NEPHROLOGY RESEARCH AND CLINICAL DEVELOPMENTS

HEMODIALYSIS

INDICATIONS, PROCEDURES AND COMPLICATIONS

NEPHROLOGY RESEARCH AND CLINICAL DEVELOPMENTS

Additional books in this series can be found on Nova's website under the Series tab.

Additional e-books in this series can be found on Nova's website under the e-book tab.

NEPHROLOGY RESEARCH AND CLINICAL DEVELOPMENTS

HEMODIALYSIS

INDICATIONS, PROCEDURES AND COMPLICATIONS

YURI F. CABRAL
AND
MARINA COSTA DE SANTOS
EDITORS

Nova Science Publishers, Inc.
New York

Library of Congress Cataloging-in-Publication Data

Library of Congress Control Number 2012933662

ISBN: 978-1-62081-301-0

Published by Nova Science Publishers, Inc. † New York

Contents

Preface

In this book, the authors present topical research in the study of the indications, procedures and complications of hemodialysis. Topics discussed in this compilation include cardiovascular involvement in chronic kidney disease; nutritional therapy during hemodialysis; vascular access and common complications in patients undergoing hemodialysis treatment; prevention of hemodialysis catheter-related infections; antiplatelet medication and the risk of bleeding in hemodialysis; and vascular calcifications in end stage renal disease.

Chapter I - Cardiovascular disease is leading cause of morbidity and mortality in CKD patients; cardiovascular risk increases since early stages of CKD because of association with other major cardiovascular risk factors, such as diabetes, hypertension or both.

Cardiovascular damage is primary substained by atherosclerotic damage due to chronic inflammatory status of CKD patients together with calcium – phosphorus imbalance and secondary hyperparathyroidism.

Chapter II - Dialysis can worsen the nutritional status of dialysis patients and malnutrition worsens treatment prognosis. Hence, specific and personal nutritional therapy, with proper food intake, has a decisive role on the positive prognosis of chronic kidney disease patients undergoing hemodialysis. This chapter will cover the metabolic changes caused by chronic kidney disease which serve to guide appropriate nutritional therapy. The nutritional recommendations for the chronic kidney disease patient undergoing hemodialysis will be approached by their historical aspect and under the light of the current consensus and controversies. Assuming that appropriate food intake is challenging for the patient and for the healthcare team, the chapter will present a discussion on the etiological factors of inappropriate food intake by hemodialysis patients and the current strategies for overcoming this difficulty. Finally, the chapter will cover the perspectives and innovations of nutritional therapy during hemodialysis in order to improve food intake and the quality of life of hemodialysis patients.

Chapter III - Despite the widespread use of peritoneal dialysis and renal transplantation, hemodialysis remains the main renal replacement therapy in most countries worldwide. Hemodialysis is required in three general situations: acute renal failure, end-stage renal disease and poisonings. Successful hemodialysis in any of these settings requires access to large blood vessels capable of supporting rapid extracorporeal blood flow. Central venous catheters are the preffered vascular access for patients presenting with acute renal failure and for chronic end-stage renal disease patients without permanent arteriovenous access or with failed vascular access. Adequate and timely preparation of vascular access in patients with chronic kidney disease stage 4 (estimated glomerular filtration rate below 30 ml per min per 1,73 m^2) can decrease morbidity and perhaps mortality. The access should generally be placed in the nondominant upper extremity. Venipuncture should therefore be restricted to the arm not chosen for eventual access placement so that the veins in the other arm will be preserve. There are a number of clinical indications to initiate dialysis in patients with acute renal failure or end-stage renal disease. These include: pericarditis or pleuritis (urgent indication), progressive uremic encephalopathy or neuropathy, with signs such as confusion, asterixis, tremor, multifocal myoclonus, wrist or foot drop, or, in severe cases, seizures (urgent indication), a clinically significant bleeding diathesis attributable to uremia (urgent indication), fluid overload refractory to diuretics, hypertension poorly responsive to antihypertensive medications, persistent metabolic disturbances that are refractory to medical therapy - hyperkalemia, metabolic acidosis, hypercalcemia, hypocalcemia, and hyperphosphatemia, persistent nausea and vomiting, evidence of malnutrition. Relative indications for the initiation of dialysis include decreased attentiveness and cognitive tasking, depression, persistent pruritus or the restless leg syndrome. Usually dialysis is initiated in adult patients with chronic kidney disease when the estimated glomerular filtration rate decrease to about 10 mL per minute per 1.73 m^2.

Multiple modalities of renal replacement therapy are currently available. These include intermittent hemodialysis, hemofiltration and hemodiafiltration, continuous renal replacement therapies, and hybrid therapies, such as sustained low-efficiency dialysis. Continuous renal replacement therapies represents a family of continuous modalities that provide support for severely ill patients with acute renal failure.

The most common acute complications during hemodialysis treatments are hypotension, hypertension, cramps, nausea and vomiting, headache, chest pain, back pain, itching. These complications are generally caused by multiple underlying mechanisms and are poorly understood.

This chapter will review indications, vascular access, different modalities and common and less common complications in patients undergoing hemodialysis treatment.

Chapter IV - Despite all efforts to reduce the use of catheters in hemodialysis patients because of related complications, the frequency of catheter use continues to rise. Almost 30% of chronic hemodialysis patients are dependent on central venous catheters (CVC) for their vascular access. CVC have significantly higher rates of infection when compared to grafts and fistulae. It has been estimated that the relative risk for infection in tunneled catheters, cuffed, and uncuffed, when compared with native arteriovenous fistulae is 15.5 and 22.5, respectively. Ideally, dialysis centers should have a catheter-related bacteremia rate of less than 1 per 1000 catheter-days. The most important risk factors for catheter-related infections (CRI) include the presence of diabetes, peripheral atherosclerosis, a previous history of bacteremia, nasal carriage of *Staphylococcus aureus*, longer duration of catheter use, and local infection. CRI is an important source of morbidity and mortality in hemodialysis patients, being responsible for the deaths of approximately 2000 to 5000 hemodialysis patients each year in the United States. A recent clinical trial addressing the prevention of CRI demonstrated that 12% of bacteremia episodes resulted in death. The costs to the health care system are also substantial. Data from the United States Renal Data System and Medicare estimated the total costs of CRI may approach 1 billion dollars per year. Several techniques have been used to decrease the incidence of CRI. These include the use of systemic antibiotics around the time of catheter placement, antimicrobial lock solutions, antimicrobial impregnated catheters, exit-site antimicrobials, and agents used to reduce nasal colonization. The main health risks associated with antimicrobial interventions include side effects such as ototoxicity with gentamicin, hypocalcaemia with citrate, and possible emergence of resistant organisms. These interventions also entail additional costs to the health care provider. This review describes the epidemic problem of CRI, and reviews recent clinical trials of antimicrobial interventions for the prevention of CRI and the importance of strict infection prophylaxis protocol based on universal precautions against infection.

Chapter V - More than 530,000 patients develop end stage renal disease every year in the United States, vast majority requiring hemodialysis (HD). This procedure has become much safer now with the improved water treatments, advent of better dialysis equipment and safety protocols followed during dialysis. However, this procedure still has many complications and adverse events associated with it, most of which occur in the acute setting. The most common complication is hypotension.

Chapter VI - In hemodialysis patients, antiplatelet medications are used in various situations which include prevention of ischemic and thrombotic complications. The recent rapid increase in the number of hemodialysis patients due to diabetes mellitus and advanced age of patients has resulted in an increased demand for percutaneous intervention or coronary artery bypass grafting requiring long-term adjunctive antiplatelet or anticoagulant medications. Patients with chronic kidney disease, particularly hemodialysis patients, are at high risk of bleeding, and long-term antiplatelet therapy in hemodialysis patients may result in harmful bleeding. Despite this situation, the influence of antiplatelet therapy on bleeding in hemodialysis patients has not been sufficiently studied. We investigated bleeding events that required the cessation of the use of heparin for hemodialysis in all the hemodialysis patients treated in our clinic. During the treatment in our clinic, 21 of 52 patients with antiplatelet therapy experienced a bleeding event (gastrointestinal bleeding 16, brain stem hemorrhage 2, others 3), while 7 of 59 patients without antiplatelet therapy had a bleeding event (gastrointestinal bleeding 7) ($p<0.001$). It's worth noting that, the diabetic patients with antiplatelet therapy had the highest incidence of bleeding events. Among the patients with antiplatelet therapy, no correlations were found between bleeding events and the duration of antiplatelet therapy and the number of agents.

Our results showed that antiplatelet therapy can induce bleeding events more frequently in hemodialysis patients, especially in diabetic patients, than in non-hemodialysis patients, and antiplatelet therapy should be given only under prudent consideration of the associated risks and benefits.

Chapter VII - Vascular calcifications (VCs) are more frequent and severe in patients with CKD on dialysis than in subjects from the general population. Both high phosphorus and positive calcium balance from calcium-containing phosphate binders are considered as strong responsible factors of vascular calcification process and adverse events. Therefore, guidelines recommend limiting the use of calcium containing phosphate binders in presence of known vascular and or valvular calcifications in CKD patients not yet on dialysis. We describe our experience on vascular calcification in dialysis patients. These results indicated that CAC could represent a step in the continuum of events responsible for the CV mortality in CKD-5.

In: Hemodialysis: Indications, Procedures and Complications ISBN: 978-1-62081-301-0
Editors: Y F. Cabral and M. Costa De Santos

Chapter I

Cardiovascular Involvement in Chronic Kidney Disease

***Luca Di Lullo*[1], *Fulvio Floccari*[2], *Rodolfo Rivera*[2] *and Antonio Granata*[4]**
[1]Colleferro, Italy
[2]Civitavecchia, Italy
[3]Monza, Italy
[4]Agrigento, Italy

Epidemiology

1. Introduction

Cardiovascular disease is leading cause of morbidity and mortality in CKD patients; cardiovascular risk increases since early stages of CKD because of association with other major cardiovascular risk factors, such as diabetes, hypertension or both [1].

Cardiovascular damage is primary substained by atherosclerotic damage due to chronic inflammatory status of CKD patients together with calcium – phosphorus imbalance and secondary hyperparathyroidism.

1.1. Dialysis

In hemodialysis patients cardiovascular disease is accounting for 45% of deaths and about 20% of cardiac deaths are linked to coronary heart disease and myocardial infarction. High cardiovascular mortality rate is well illustrated by comparing cardiovascular mortality rates in general population and hemodialysis patients in which mortality rates are 10 to 30% higher independently from age and sex. This is particularly due to increased cardiovascular comorbidities before starting hemodialysis therapy: about 40% patients show diagnosis of chronic coronary disease, 40 % have congestive heart failure, 20% have peripheral vascular disease and 10% have had strokes or transient ischemic attacks [2].

1.2. Pre – Dialysis

Undoubtely, presence of cardiovascular damage before starting renal replacement therapy points up on incident cardiovascular comorbities since early stages of chronic kidney disease. Patients with CrCl above 50 ml/min present less incidence of left ventricular hypertrophy in respect of those patients with CrCl under 25 ml/min. Patients with CKD show higher prevalence of coronary artery disease and heart failure compared to normal population [3].

Patients with CKD present rates of cardiovascular events next to 102 per 1000 patients/year [4].

2. Risk Factors

Cardiovascular risk factors are usually classified as traditional and non - traditional; first ones are defined as those conferring increased cardiovascular risk in general population and they include age, diabetes and hypertension, all prevalent in CKD patients.

Non – traditional cardiovascular risk factors refer to those increased as kidney function declines: there are postulated as typical of these patients population (see Table 1).

Most of risk factors lead to atherosclerotic damage, arteriosclerosis and cardiomyopathy with consequent development of ischemic heart disease and heart failure. Dyslipidemia and hyperhomocysteinemia may contribute to atherosclerotic damage progression such as calcium – phosphorus product imbalancement and secondary hyperparathyroidism vascular impact.

2.1. Traditional Risk Factors

2.1.1. Blood Pressure

Hypertension may be cause and effect of kidney disease and more of 70% of stage 1 CKD patients are hypertensive with prevalence strictly related to glomerular filtration rate decline. At the start of hemodialysis treatment, almost 90% of patients present blood pressures above 145/90 mmHg [5].

Increased adverse cardiovascular events and mortality are evident when post – dialysis systolic blood pressure is above 180 mmHg and hypertension is often under treated in hemodialysis patients [6].

Table 1.

TRADITIONAL RISK FACTORS	NON – TRADITIONAL RISK FACTORS
Age	Albuminuria
Male gender	Hyperhomocysteinemia
Hypertension	Anemia
Higher LDL – C	Abnormal calcium/phosphate product
Lower HDL – C	Extracellular fluid volume overload
Diabetes	Electrolyte imbalance
Smoking	Oxidative stress
Menopause	Chronic inflammation
Physical inactivity	Malnutrition
Left ventricular hypertrophy	Altered nitric oxide/endothelin balance
Familiar history of cardiovascular diease	Sleep disturbances

On the other hand, patients (especially hemodialysis patients) often present low blood pressures that can be associated with other comorbidities such as heart failure and pericardial effusions. Intradialytic hypotension is quite common feature and it can be identified as an independent risk factor for cardiovascular outcome [7].

Hypertension is therefore highly prevalent in CKD patients not on dialysis; data from literature show as 80% of patients with CrCl below 75 ml/min are hypertensive ones [8].

Hypertension represents an independent risk factor for cardiovascular outcomes both in diabetic and non diabetic patients.

2.1.2. Dyslipidemia

Since early stages of CKD patients often present diabetes and hypertension frequently associated to LDL Cholesterol increase. An associated nephrotic syndrome can worse dyslipidemic pattern. HDL Cholesterol is often reduced while triglycerides are usually elevated [9].

About 50% of hemodialysis patients present LDL – C levels over 100 mg/dL, while this prevalence rise up to 70% in peritoneal dialysis patients.

On the other hand, as hemodialysis treatment goes on, patients often reveal hypocholesterolemia, a malnutrition index often associated with low serum albumin and elevated levels of C- reactive protein (CRP) [10].

2.1.3. Diabetes Mellitus

Presence of diabetes mellitus in dialysis patients represent an independent risk factor for ischemic heart disease and heart failure. Diabetic dialysis patients often present worse prognosis linked to sub – optimal therapeutical regimen schemes.

Diabetes, together with arterial hypertension, is the most common cause of chronic kidney disease and microalbuminuria is first clinical manifestation of diabetic nephropathy [11].

2.1.4. Left Ventricular Hypertrophy (LVH)

LVH, high prevalent in Stage 3 and stage 4 CKD patients, is resulting from pressure and volume overload. Blood pressure overload is due to hypertension, valvular heart disease and atherosclerosis [12]. Valvular heart disease often depends from secondary hyperparathyroidism and calcium – phosphorus product imbalancement. On the other hand, volume overload refers to anemia, increased extracellular volume and vascular access hemodynamic effects [13].

Initially, LVH is a concentric one with uniform increase in left ventricular wall thickness from pressure overload. As kidney failure goes on, volume overload gives raise to an eccentric LVH with increased left ventricular diameters and proportional increase in left ventricular wall thickness [13].

As LVH proceeds, capillary density decreases and perfusion goes down leading to fibrotic involution of myocardial architecture [14].

Pre – dialysis population shows LVH prevalence from 20 to 50 %, while echocardiographic findings reveal LVH prevalence of about 70 % in dialysis patients [14].

2.2. Non - Traditional Risk Factors

2.2.1. Homocysteine

Homocysteine has been indicated as cardiovascular risk factor both in general population (especially as myocardial infarction and stroke risk factor), and CKD patients.

Hemodialysis patients present raised homocysteine levels linked to progressive decline of kidney function. Some studies have considered hyperhomocysteinemia as an independent risk factor for cardiovascular mortality in dialysis patients. [15].

It's important to underline that homocysteine levels are linked to nutritional status of patients, often associated to low plasmatic levels of folates, vitamin B_{12} and vitamin B_6 [15].

Treatment with high dosage of folic acid and B vitamins may normalize homocysteine levels but this is not completely true in hemodialysis patients.

2.2.2. Oxidant Stress and Inflammation

Oxidant stress may be defined as an imbalance between oxidants and anti – oxidants molecules. In CKD patients inflammation, malnutrition, uremic toxins and hemodialysis treatment itself can increase oxidant stress in hemodialysis population [16].

CKD patients (both pre – dialysis and dialysis) present low levels of antioxidant agents, such as glutathione [16].

There is strong association between oxidant stress and bad cardiovascular outcomes in hemodialysis patients also linked to oxidant stress impact on anemia and malnutrition. Chronic inflammation and oxidant stress may also lead to increased production of oxidized LDL with pro – atherogenic action [17].

Statin and antioxidant therapy (i.e. vitamin E supplements) can provide to control oxidant stress in CKD patients but results are still to be confirmed [9].

Left Heart Failure and Chronic Kidney Disease

1. Introduction

Left ventricular hypertrophy (LVH) is common in almost 40% patient with mild to moderate chronic kidney disease to raise up to 70% in patients starting hemodialysis treatment [18]. Both forms (concentric and eccentric) could be present, often associated, leading to increased mortality and morbidity risk.

Left ventricular hypertrophy, together with other cardiovascular risk factors (tobacco use, hypertension, diabetes mellitus, anemia), contributes to accelerate towards left heart failure [18].

Once starting hemodialysis treatment, only 15 – 20% of patients show normal echocardiographic patterns, while up to 15% of patients already present echocardiographic aspect of left ventricular disfunction [19] (Figure 1).

Changes in left ventricle geometry could refer to chronic volume overload in these patients, especially in end stage CKD patients on hemodialysis or peritoneal dialysis treatment [20].

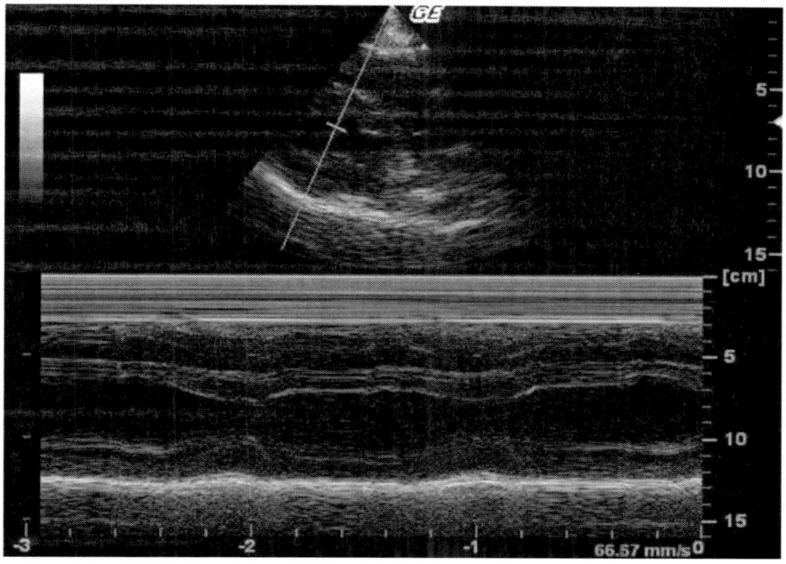

Figure 1. Left ventricular hypertrophy in end – stage kidney disease.

As a result, it becomes clear that we assist to shift from concentric hypertrophy with normal left ventricular volumes to an eccentric hypertrophy with dilation of left ventricle.

Eccentric LVH determines an impairment both sistolic and diastolic function of left ventricle that leads to myocardial disfunction and decrease in myocardial contractility [21].

2. Pathophysiology

LVH represent an adaptive process in response to chronic volume and pressure overload to left heart chambers and consequent increase in myocardial work. Increase in volume and pressure overload is often accompanied with local secretion of neurohormones, growth factors and vasoactive cytokines [22].

As myocardial stress increases, myocardial energy expenditure and oxygen consumption increase in the same way until to stress myocardial cells that have to work against raised pressures and volumes [22].

Initial effects of LVH are beneficial because it becomes possible to generate higher intraventricular pressures without increasing parietal stress; these changes can be observed in physiological condition also as late pregnancy, after intensive training in athletes or normal growth to adulthood [23].

Initial LVH is an adaptive status in which pressure and volume overload lead only to myocardial cells hyperplasia without any functional damage [24].

Pathophysiological picture changes if hypertrophic process goes on and myocardial stress couples with over – stretching of papillary muscles, oxidant stress, apoptosis and increase in extracellular matrix until to myocardial fibrosis [25].

Consequences are electrophysiological abnormalities and left diastolic function impairment to maintain systolic efficiency [26].

Pressure and volume overloads in CKD patients are now known as hemodynamic risk factors. Pressure overload results from increase in left ventricle afterload as we observe in hypertensive status, atherosclerosis and valvular stenosis, such as aortic stenosis [25, 26].

Volume overload belong to increased extracellular volume, anemia and venous preload due to presence of vascular access in hemodialysis patients [25].

As we discussed above, concentric hypertrophy is an adaptive process to chronic pressure overload on left ventricle. Result is an addition of new muscular tissue with an increase in myocyte thickness [25, 26].

Increased left ventricular mass means increased thickness of interventricular septum and posterior wall [24, 25, 26]

Eccentric hypertrophy is an adaptive mechanism too in response to chronic volume overload. Left ventricle volume overload give new impulse to addition of new sarcomeres [26]

As consequence, increased left ventricular mass in associated with increased left ventricular volume and posterior wall thickness.

Together with pressure and volume overload, neurohormonal factors and other cytokines may contribute to LVH: natriuretic peptides, troponin, homocysteine, ADMA, endhotelin, catecholamine and high sympathetic activity [26].

3. Pathology

Autoptic findings in end stage CKD heart patients are characterized by enlarged chambers' size, thickened walls and marked left ventricular hypertrophy.

Light microscopy reveals myocytes hypertrophy with hyperplasia of non – myocytic components. Coronary arteries are also involved in hypertrophic process with widespread evidences of atheromatous calcific plaques and intramural calcifications [27].

A Japanese study pointed up pathophysiological process of dilated cardiomyopathy and demonstrated how myocardiocytes of end – stage CKD patients were greater than myocardiocytes from patients without kidney failure [28].

Another key point is represented by interstitial fibrosis that is a characteristic finding in CKD patients due to fibroblasts proliferation and it's more marked than in diabetic patients [29]. An additional factor contributing to fibrosis is represented by secondary hyperparathyroidism because fibrosis in hemodialysis patients. Fibroblasts proliferation PTH itself is a profibrotic agent and this is clearly underlined by widespread intramyocardial and increased matrix collagen lead to imbalance to myocyte- fibroblast ratio [31].

Left ventricular diastolic dysfunction and arrhythmias are clinical aspects of pathological damages described above; arrhythmias are probably related to slower calcium re – uptake by sarcoplasmic reticulum, delayed relaxation phase of cardiac cycle and, thus, delay of depolarization phase [32].

4. Cardiac Failure

It's quite difficult to assess left ventricle functional abnormalities in CKD patients because of absence of symptoms. Silent echocardiographic signs are evident since stage III –

IV of CKD and Stage V CKD patients present abnormal values of interventricular septum and left ventricular volumes almost at dialysis onset.

4.1. Diastolic Dysfunction

Since early stages of CKD, echocardiography shows abnormalities related to left ventricular diastolic dysfunction with an inversion of E/A ratio as measured on mitral valve Doppler examination [32].

E/A ratio inversion and refilling imbalance are more evident in hemodialysis patients and it's more evident in respect of patients with hypertensive cardiac disease, but milder than observed in patients with hypertrophic cardiomyopathy [32].

Abormal and impaired ventricular refilling in uremic patients is related to myocardial fibrosis causing increased stiffness of ventricular walls and delayed relaxation as demonstrated by electrophysiological examination [33]

Due to increased stiffness, small changes in volume also can result in larger changes in left ventricular pressures leading to pulmonary edema more frequently than in cardiovascular patients not affected by chronic kidney disease [32, 33].

Onset symptoms of diastolic dysfunction are also represented by symptomatic hypotension and hemodynamic instability because of volume depletion during hemodialysis session that results in significant fall of left ventricular pressure.

4.2. Systolic Disfunction

Systolic function is usually normal in patients with advanced chronic kidney disease without any cardiologic clinical antecedent.

Clinical findings related to an impaired systolic function can be observed in CKD patients with cardiac involvement and in long – term hemodialysis patients with chronic hemodynamic overload [19, 34].

First of all, myocardial contractility depression can represent final pathway of any king of cardiomiopathy with significant volume overload. This is worse clinical condition and show bad long – term prognosis in respect of all clinical conditions (such as arterial hypertension) characterized by concentric hypertrophy or eccentric hypertrophy with normal systolic function [34].

Hemodialysis patients also present a chronic coronary heart disease as primum movens of systolic dysfunction. Laboratory findings have shown that uremic toxins can be reduce contraction strength of myocardiocytes in culture [35].

It has also been shown that renal transplantation can normalize systolic function of previous hemodialyzed patients but cannot affect left ventricle mass index.

4.3. Symptomatic Heart Failure

Heart failure represent clinical condition in which heart cannot provide sufficient output for metabolic needs at rest.

Left ventricular hypertrophy, if not treated, could be first step towards development of clinical heart failure. In Canadian population study, after performing echocardiography at time 0 and after one year of hemodialysis treatment, it was postulated that an increase of left ventricular mass index and decrease of shoretening fraction were independent risk factor for developing of heart failure [36].

Table 2. Executive summary dal "World Symposium on Primary Pulmonary Hypertension". Rich S. Editor. http//www.who.int/ncd/cvd/pph.html

1 – Clinical Classification of Pulmonary Arterial Hypertension.
1.1 – Idiopatic pulmonary arterial hypertension.
• Sporadic. • Familiar.
1.2 – Pulmonary arterial hypertension associated with:
• Connective tissue disease. • Congenital heart disease. • Portal hypertension. • HIV infection. • Anorexigens and other toxic drugs. • Persistent pulmonary hypertension of the newborn.
2 – Pulmonary venous hypertension.
2.1 – Left – sided atrial or ventricular heart disease. 2.2 – Extrinsic compression of central pulmonary veins. 2.3 – Pulmonary veno – occlusion disease.
3 – Pulmonary Hyoertension associated with disorders of respiratory system and/or hypoxemia.
3.1 – Chronic obstructive pulmonary disease. 3.2 – Interstitial lung disease. 3.3 – Sleep – disordered breathing. 3.4 – Chronic exposure to high altitude. 3.5 – Cystic fibrosis.
4 – Pulmonary hypertension due to chronic thrombotic and/or embolic disease.
4.1 – Thromboembolic obstruction of proximal pulmonary arteries. 4.2 – Thromboembolic obstruction of distal pulmonary arteries. • Pulmonary embolism. • "In situ" thrombosis. • Thalassemia.
5 – Pulmonary hypertension due to disorders directly affecting pulmonary vasculature.
5.1 – Inflammatory disease.
• Schistosomiasis / Sarcoidosis.
5.2 – Pulmonary capillary hemangiomatosis.

Table 3. WHO Functional Classification of Pulmonary Hypertension

CLASS I	Patients without limitation of physical activity. Ordinary physical activity does not cause undue dyspnea or fatigue, chest pain or syncope.
CLASS II	Patients with slight limitation of physical activity. They are confartable at rest. Ordinary physical activity causes undue dyspnea or fatigue, chest pain or near syncope.
CLASS III	Patients with marked limitation of physical activity. They are confartable at rest. Less than ordinary activity causes undue dyspnea or fatigue, chest pain or near syncope.
CLASS IV	Patients with inability to carry out any physical activity without symptoms. Patients manifest signs of right heart failure. Dyspnea and/or fatigue may even be present at rest. Discomfort is increased by any physical activity.

Therefore systolic dysfunction can provide ultrastructural abnormalities on muscle fiber length and end diastolic volume together with accelerated sympathetic activity, enhanced secretion of neurohormones (angiotensin II, vasopressin, endhotelin, BNP and ANP) and abnormal production of ouabain – like mediators aging on Na – K ATPasi channels: final result is an enhanced contractility together with an impaired relaxation [37].

Clinical onset is typical with dyspnea and pulmonary venous congestion 'till pulmonary edema often worsened by an underlying hypertrophic cardiomiopathy.

Pulmonary Hypertension and Right Heart Failure in Chronic Kidney Disease

1. Introduction

Pulmonary hypertension is described as an increased sistolic pulmonary pressure above 30 mmHg. Primary pulmonary hypertension represent an uncommon clinical diagnosis with a 2 for million cases prevalence all over the world. Table 2 shows clinical classification of Pulmonary Hypertension as it was proposed by World Symposium on Pulmonary Hypertension and confirmed by WHO. Table 3 shows functional classification of Pulmonary Hypertension.

In CKD patients available data report 40% prevalence of pulmonary hypertension in hemodialysis patients, 10% in peritoneal dialysis patients and pre – dialysis patients [38]. At the same time, right ventricular dysfunction assessment in hemodialysis patients is more effective if performed by TAPSE evaluation.

Recently published data reported as about 20% hemodialysis patients with AFV show abnormal TAPSE values (<15 mm), while CVC carriers present normal ones [39].

In chronic hemodialysis patients presence of an artero – venous shunt, as it happens with an artero – venous fistula, involves preload increase on right heart chambers with adverse potential long – term effects on their performance.

These patients often show right ventricular and atrial volumes next to maximum allowed (and above) before hemodialysis treatment to come back in normal ranges at the end of dialysis treatment according to reduction of extracellular fluid volumes.

Together with described above, we attend to reduction of left ventricular telediastolic volume with concomitant increasing of ejection fraction that point up beneficial effects of hemodialysis therapy on cardiac performance.

Otherwise, at present time, there are not significant clinical data about CKD patients on pre – dialysis; at the same it is possible to say that it's common to observe abnormalities of right ventricular function echocardiographic parameters before those linked to left ventricular systolic function parameters.

Some patients without any pulmonary comorbidity (BPCI, Pulmonary Fibrosis) can show TAPSE index reduction and increased atrio – ventricular volumes and pressures when their diastolic left ventricular parameters (E/A ratio) are still in normal ranges.

2. Pathophysiology

Pathophysiology of secondary pulmonary hypertension in CKD patients is still complex and not clear. We certainly observe pulmonary circulation impairment together with chronic volume overload, connective tissue diseases, acquired and congenital cardiopathies, HIV syndrome, hepatic cirrhosis with portal hypertension and all chronic comorbidities with increased pressures in left heart side. CKD patients present two characteristic clinical features: anemia and (in most of them) artero – venous fistula; both factors lead to increased pre – load on right heart chambers. [38].

Pulmonary hypertension could lead to increased levels of cytokines and growth factors, such as FGF, PDGF and TGF- β with concomitant pulmonary ACE activation. As consequence we assist to abnormal smooth muscle cells proliferation until fibrosis.

Endhotelial dysfunction, together with lower activation of NOS, increased levels of serum endhotelin and fibrin storages, could involve an extensive growth of endhotelial cells until complete obliteration of pulmonary vessels.

Mio – intimal proliferation, intimal laminated (both concentric and eccentric) fibrosis, thrombosis and arterial obliteration are typical pathological features of disease progression.

Nephrologists have to remember that right ventricle has thin muscle equipment because it usually works with low blood pressure unable to force high vascular resistenze.

Pulmonary hypertension derived pressure overload, once right heart chambers loss their distensibility, leads to tricuspidal regurgitation and further right heart volume overload.

3. Diagnosis

Pulmonary hypertension has no patognomonic and distinctive symptoms and signs. At the onset, we usually observe mild to moderate dyspnea (80% of patients), fatigue, hypotensive crisis and Reynaud phenomenon. These clinical findings are usually observed in CKD patients also and nephrologists could undervalue secondary pulmonary hypertension diagnosis.

Systolic pulmonary pressure evaluation is easily performed by standard trans – thoracic echocardiography. AHA and SIEC guidelines collect it among essential parameters to investigate in basic echocardiography.

Preliminary B- Mode echocardiography, however, allows to detect some ultrasound aspects could suggest pulmonary hypertension:

1. Right heart chamber dilation;
2. "D" shape of right ventricle by flattening of interventricular septum;
3. Absence of inferior vena cava inhalatory collapse.

M- Mode view will show small or absent "a" (atrial) wave.

Diagnostic accuracy of these echocardiographic findings is quite poor, both for specificity and sensibility. Therefore, they're all qualitative features and they don't allow both to evaluate right ventricular impairment degree and response to pharmacological therapy.

It becames crucial to complete our echocardiographic test with Doppler evaluation; pulmonary arterial pressure is performed by tricuspidal and pulmonary regurgitation speed assay.

Tricuspidal regurgitation speed (V_{TR}) is evaluated by four chambers echocardiographic apical view with ultrasound probe following trans – valvular flow to catch regurgitation volume.

La V_{TR} points up systolic pressure gradient between two right heart sections. If we add right atrial pressure, we obtain right ventricle systolic pressure (PAPs)

PAPs = 4 (VTR)2 + RAP (right atrial pressure)

Right atrial pressure can be estimated on basic trans – thoracic echocardiography with inhalatory collapse in VCI diameter. When VCI diameter goes down more 50% with inhalation, right atrium pressure is lower than 10 mmHg; if VCI inhalatory collapse is lower than 50%, right atrium pressure is higher than 10 mmHg. Therefore, if right atrium is dilated (area > 15 cm^2), RAP is 15 mmHg at least.

It's important to underline that all we have discussed above became avoid if we are in presence of pulmonary valve stenosis or any other mechanical obstruction to right ventricle outflow.

Pulmonary hypertension is characterized by tricuspidal regurgitation speed $\geq$ 2 m/s (normal value is lower than 1 m/s)

Telediastolic speed of pulmonary regurgitation represent tele diastolic pressure gradient between pulmonary artery and right ventricle. At the end of diastole, right ventricular pressure should be the same of right atrial pressure:

PAEDP = 4 * VPR 2 + RAP

where PAEDP is tele diastolic pulmonary arterial pressure.

Pulmonary arterial pressure is usually increased in patients with high left ventricle inflow pressures; pulse – wave Doppler study on mitral valve allow to identify restrictive pattern of trans – mitralic flow (increase of E wav, decrease of A wave and deceleration time of E wave, E/A ratio > 2).

Patients affected by portal hypertension show peculiar aspects at Doppler evaluation of sovra – hepatic veins with a well rendered retrograde flow. A wave due to increased diastolic pressure and decreased compliance of right ventricular wall.

Right ventricular function is often assessed by measuring cranio – caudale excursion capability of tricupispal valve annulus during ventricular systole (Tricuspid Annulus Plane Systolic Excursion, TAPSE). TAPSE index can be easily evaluated on M-Mode echocardiography without referring to tissue Doppler and holds good riproducibilità among echocardiographic physicians (Figure 2).

Compliant right ventricle allows wide excursion of tricuspidal annulus, while it's prevented or strongly restricted in progressive right heart impairment and failure. TAPSE is well related with diastolic function of right ventricle and blood inflow towards right atrium. TAPSE also represent good prognostic marker to stratify cardiovascular risk and it's not affected by heart rate and rhytmn. Thus, TAPSE can be also performed in patients with tachycardia or atrial fibrillation in which diastolic function evaluation is prevented by only one atrial wave on trans – mitralic Doppler. TAPSE scoring also represent a cardiovascular prognostic index together with NYHA classification.

In our experience once hemodialysis session does not affect PAPs, while significantly decrease TAPSE value as consequence of volume overload reduction following ultrafiltration, not related to myocardial stunning hypothesis because ejection fraction grow up after hemodialysis session [39].

Our results seems to sustain those of Beigi et al both about artero – venous fistulae long – term effects on cardiac output and pulmonary circulation, both with epidemiological data about prevalence of pathological PAPs values [40].

4. Management

First of all, patients with pulmonary hypertension diagnosis take benefits from lifestyle changes such as suppression of smoking and starting of mild physical practice.

As nephrologists we have to take care to good pressure control, optimal and stable hemoglobin levels and proper management of dry weight.

For whom to concern pharmacological treatment, scientific evidences and literature references have focused on digoxin, diuretics and calcium – channel blockers.

Digoxin can exert favorable hemodynamic effect when given acutely to patients with right ventricular failure from pulmonary hypertension. Further evidences show how digoxin could induce a drop off of noradrenalin circulating levels, one of biochemical agents involved in pulmonary hypertension develop and progression.

Digital - derived drugs employment has to strickly monitored in CKD patients, especially hemodialysis ones, with recurrent sampling of digoxin, heart rate and ECG evaluation [41].

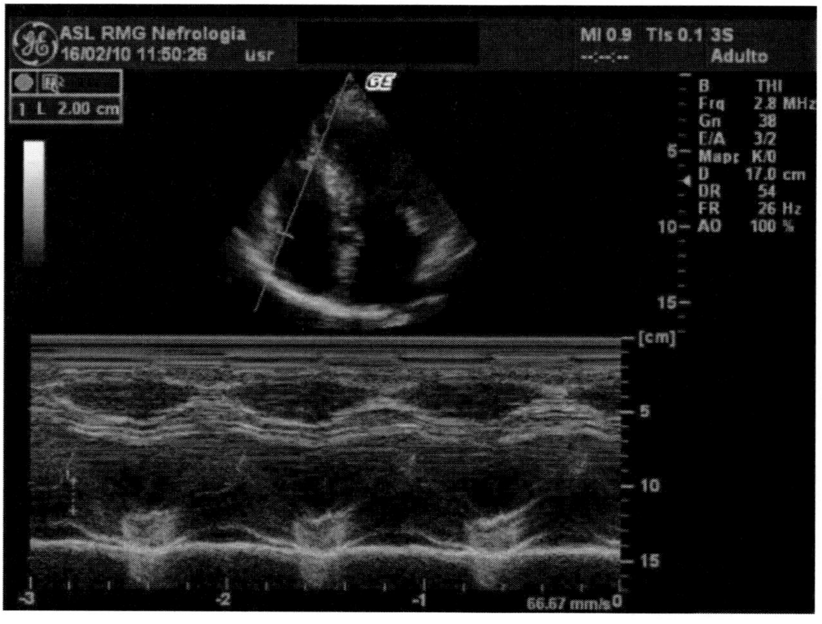

Figure 2. M- Mode Echocardiography on long – axis parasternal view: TAPSE index evaluation (in Figure 1 normal TAPSE value of 20 mm).

Volume overload represent crucial step in pathophysiological pathways to pulmonary hypertension. Loop diuretics, thiazides and aldosterone antagonists can be helpful in reducing volume overload in patients with effective diuresis, paying attention to serum potassium levels [42].

Extracorporeal ultrafiltration represent precious tool for nephrologists giving them further chances to team up with other physicians.

Oral anticoagulants employment is recommended in pulmonary hypertensive patients as underlined by retrospective data from Mayo Clinic collected in patients in whom calcium channel blockers therapy failed. Patients underwent warfarin treatment showed 91% one year and 47% three years survival rates versus 62% and 31% of patients who didn't undergo on warfarin therapy. Recommended doses were similar to those employed in venous thromboembolism profilaxys (INR between 2 and 3) [43,44].

Low molecular weight heparin represent valid alternative because of its inhibitory effects on smooth muscle cells proliferation.

Because of early reports showing reduction in pulmonary artery pressure following acute administration of vasodilators agents, it was presumed that they could be gold standard in treating PPH patients.

Common pathway by which vasodilators work could be found in reduction of intracellular calcium in vascular smooth muscle cell; therefore, most vasodilators possess growth inhibitory properties of smooth muscle cells in culture.

Among vasodilators, calcium – channel blockers have widest spread but some pharmacological properties, such as a negative inotropic effect on right ventricular function and reflex sympathetic stimulation, can worse underlying pulmonary hypertension and increasing resting heart rate.

On the other hand, it has been reported that 10 to 20 percent of PHH patients, treated with high doses of calcium channel blockers, may exhibit dramatic reduction in pulmonary arterial pressure and pulmonary vascular resistance. Patient's quality of life was restored with improved functional class and increased rate of survival [45].

Prostaglandin analogues involve many pharmacological agents helpful in modulating arterial pulmonary resistances. Among them *Epoprostenol* [46] has been shown to improve quality of life and symptoms PPH related, exercise tolerance, hemodynamics and survival rates because of vasodilators and antithrombotic effects and related effects in normalizing cardiac output.

Continuos administration through central venous catheter and therapy related side effects (CVC and exit site infections, flushing, headache, nausea, diarrhea) have limited widespread use of epoprostenol.

Trepostinil is a prostacyclin analog quite similar to epoprostenol stable at room temperature, neutral ph with a longer half – life (3 – 4 hours). In a large randomized trial, trepostinil was effective in increasing distance walking, improving exercise tolerance and reducing dyspnea. It can be administered through continuos subcutaneous infusion without needing of CVC insertion [47].

Iloprost, another prostacyclin analog, has been utilized by inhalation showing to have an acute hemodynamic effect quite similar to nitric oxide. Chronic administration leads to patients' improvement in exercise and pulmonary hemodynamics [48].

Beraprost: is a prostacyclin orally analog that have been tested in randomized double – blind controller multicentric trials showing to involve improved exercise capacity and symptoms relief, such as dyspnea at rest. Beraprost is associated with frequent side effects as headache, flushing and diarrhea [49] which limited high doses administration.

Bosentan is an endothelin receptor blocker able to improve exercise tolerance and pulmonary hemodynamics. Recommended dosage is 125 mg twice a day in PPH patients with functional class III - IV [50].

Phosphodiesterase-5 inhibitors (Vardenafil and Sildenafil) can produce pulmonary vasodilation by enhancing sustained levels of cGMP and nitric oxide.

Safety and long – term efficacy of these drugs are currently under further investigation [51].

5. Further Perspectives

Pulmonary hypertension is common and pernicious clinical condition in CKD stage 3 – 5 patients [52 – 57]. Vascular access choice and dry weight management can modify natural history of disease and nephrologists have to keep all know – how about patients' pulmonary pressures and related pharmacological treatments.

Preliminary data seems to display clear trend to early right ventricular impairment even in early stages of chronic kidey disease [58].

Proper management of nephropathy should pay attention to right ventricular performance as it could represent new challenge for cardionephrologists in 21st century.

Pericardial Disease and Chronic Kidney Disease

1. Introduction

Pericardium is composed by two layers: the visceral pericardium, a serous membrane composed by single layer of mesothelial cells adherent to the epicardial surface of the heart, and the parietal pericardium that is fibrous, about 2 mm thick and involves most of the heart, is largely poor of mesothelial cells and essentially contains collagen and elastin. Pericardial space lies between these two layers and normally contains about 50 ml of serous fluid [59].

Pericardium may be involved in many primary and secondary diseases with wide spectrum of clinical pictures. Here we can point up upon close links between pericardial disease and chronic kidney disease.

2. Pericardial Disease and CKD

Patients with Chronic Kidney Disease may present all typical pericardial clinical entities but some of them are surely more common than others. Last decades have witnessed to a dramatic improvement in caring patients with kidney failure and uremic pericarditis (as seen in the past) is quite rare to observe. Pericardial effusion (idiopathic or secondary) is more frequent, especially in hemodialysis patients and in those patients who start renal replacement therapy in critical care conditions (i.e. patients with chronic and or acute heart failure). In CKD patients following clinical conditions can be present [60]:

a) Pericardial effusion (idiopathic or secondary).
b) Acute Pericarditis.
c) Constrictive Pericarditis.

2.1. Pericardial Effusion: Classification, Clinical Features and Diagnosis

Idiopathic pericarditis and any other clinical form of pericarditis (neoplastic, infectious, autoimmune and/or inflammatory) can provide pericardial effusion (see Table 4). Pericardial effusion are common after cardiac surgery and in non – inflammatory disease such as hypothyroidism and amyloidosis.

Patients at higher risk are HIV – infected ones and CKD patients [2], especially those on renal replacement therapy because of volume overload (hemodialysis or peritoneal dialysis patients) or immunosuppressive therapies (transplant patients).

Development of pericardial effusion is a response to inflammatory/infectious damage or is strictly linked to extracellular fluids overload (uremia, hypothyroidism). Key determinants of hemodynamic consequences of pericardial effusion are pressure levels in pericardial sac and heart ability to compensated those elevated pressures.

Pressure is depening by fluid amount and by pericardial pressure/volume ratio; pericardium has normally little volume reserve and modest amounts of effusion can exert major effects on heart compliance [61].

Table 4. Classification of pericardial disease

Idiopathic	
Infectious	Viral (echovirus, coxackievirus, adenovirus, cytomegalovirus, hepatitis B, HIV), bacterial (Pneumococcus, Staphylococcus, Streptococcus, Mycoplasma, Lyme disease, Hemophilus influenza, Neisseria Meningitidis), mycobacteria (M. Tubecolosis, M. avium), fungal (histoplasmosis, coccidiomycosis), protozoal
Immune – inflammatory	Connective tissue disease (systemic lupus erythematosus, rheumatoid arthritis, scleroderma, mixed), arteritis (polyarteritis nodosa, temporal arteritis), early post – myocardial infarction, late post – myocardial infarction, drug – induced (procainamide, hydralazine, isoniazid, cyclosporine)
Neoplastic disease	Primary: mesothelioma, fibrosarcoma. Secondary
Radiation induced	
Early post – cardiac surgery	
Device and procedure related	Coronary angioplasty, implantable devices
Trauma	Blunt and penetrating, post cardiopulmonary resuscitation
Congenital	Cysts, congenital absence
Miscellaneous	Chronic kidney disease, hypothyroidism, amyloidosis, aortic dissection

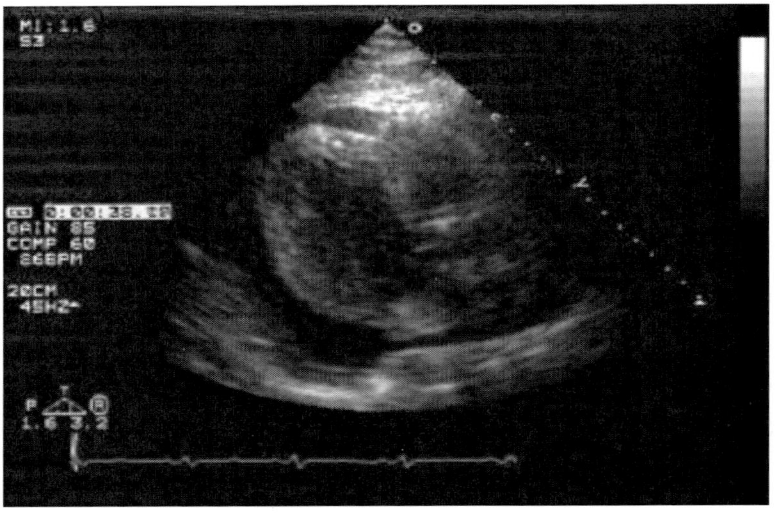

Figure 3. Mild pericardial effusion in Stage V CKD patient.

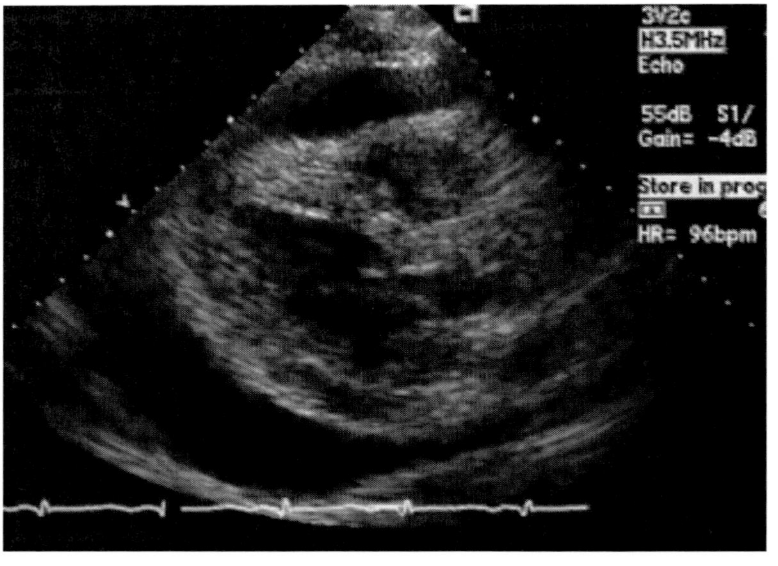

Figure 4. Severe pericardial effusion in hemodialysis patient.

Large slowly accumulating effusions are well tolerated in contrast to small acute fluid overloads.

Pericardial effusion can be classified as follows:

- MILD (posterior only pericardial effusion with width less than 1 cm) (Figure 3).
- MODERATE (all around cardiac muscle with width less than 1 cm.
- SEVERE (all around cardiac muscle with width more than 1 cm) (Figure 4).

Clinical presentation is not univocal. Occasionally, very large, asymptomatic chronic effusions are discovered only by performing chest radiography.

Many patients can present pericardial pain but, on the other hand, many others can be clinically silent 'till cardiac tamponade [61].

Usually patients with mild to moderate effusion present with dyspnea and, especially in hemodialysis patients, symptomatic hypotension.

Cardiovascular examination is usually normal except when effusion is a moderate – severe one and cardiac impulse may be difficult to palpate and heart sound muffled.

If tamponade is present, patients are uncomfortable with signs reflecting reduced cardiac output and shock such as tachypnea, diaphoresis, cool estremities, peripheral cyanosis and depressed sensorium. Hypotension is always present and paradoxical pulse is the rule, while jugular venous pressure is markedly elevated [61].

ECG shows reduced voltage and electric alternans of QRS complex; reduced QRS voltage is non – specific because it can be caused by other disease such as emphysema, myocardial disease and pneumothorax. Electric alternans is specific but insensitive for severe effusions with tamponade [62].

On chest radiography cardiac shadow remains normal until effusion is at least moderate, then lateral views can reveal separation of parietal pericardial fat from epicardium.

Echocardiography represent the gold standard to evaluate a pericardial effusion and it is performed in M – mode and B – mode allowing to discover separation (as an hypoechogenic space) between parietal and visceral pericardium.

Separations should be present for the entire cardiac cycle to be classified as effusions; small effusions are first evident on posterobasal left ventricle. As fluid increases it spreads on anterior heart, laterally and behind left atrium [63].

In modern population of hemodialysis patients clinical presentation is quite similar to acute pericarditis with chest pain, fever, leukocytosis and pericardial friction rub.

Sometimes patients present with an asymptomatic pericardial effusion causing hypotension during and after ultrafiltration session.

ECG examination often reflects high incidence of associated abnormalities like ventricular hypertrophy, previous myocardial infarction or electrolytes imbalncement (i.e. hyperkaliemia).

Chest radiography may reveal cardiac enlargement often related to volume overload, pericardial effusion or both. Asymptomatic effusion are common in hemodialysis patients and they have to be suspected in chronic hypotensive patients in which dry weight has been reached [60].

2.1.1. Management of Pericardial Effusion

Management of pericardial effusion is dictated by presence or not of cardiac tamponade.

If tamponade is not present we can face several categories of patients; some of them have acute pericarditis with mild to moderate effusion detected on routine evaluation. Some patients undergo echocardiographic examination because of other disease involving pericardium, others are totally asymptomatic and effusions are detected when diagnostic tests performed to investigate cardiovascular assessment [64].

In most of cases an etiology is well – known or is suggested by clinical history (neoplastic or autoimmune diseases, radiant therapy) and therapy is focused on primary disease.

When diagnosis is not so clear, other tests will be performed to get a more complete clinical idea on patient; skin testing for tubercolosis and screening for neoplastic or autoimmune disease and infections should be considered to start specific therapy

Patients with chronic heart failure should need more aggressive diuretic therapy in addition to chronic one, while those with autoimmune disorders usually undergo and steroid therapy [64].

Management in classic uremic pericarditis is intensive hemodialysis as well as drainage in patients with pre – tamponade or tamponade effusions.

Patients with symptomatic pericarditis always respond to the initial intensification of hemodialysis sessions but heparin should be used with care because of potential risk hemorrhagic pericarditis with tamponade.

Pericardial effusion without hemodynamic compromission usually resolves after several weeks of intensive hemodyalisis treatment [65].

In addition, NSAIDs therapy for pericardial pain is indicated avoiding corticosteroids therapy [64, 65].

2.2 Acute Pericarditis

Acute pericarditis is defined as symptoms or signs resulting from pericardial inflammation of one to two weeks duration occurring in a wide variety of disease as listed in table 1.

Most of cases are idiopathic forms with no specific etiology but many of them are supposed to have a viral etiology [61, 62].

Acute pericarditis always arises with chest pain, mimicking angina and myocardial infarction but it's not oppressive like in those cases. Pain can be severe, always pleuritic – like and sharp, with rapid onset, commonly substernal but sometimes centered at epigastric level. Sometimes it can be radiated to left arm leading to confusion with angina but it's typical radiation is to trapezius ridge.

Pain relief can be obtained by sitting forward, while it is worsened by lying down. Together with pain, dyspnea and cough can be present [64].

At physical examination, patients appear uncomfortable, anxious and may have fever and sinus tachycardia. Heart examination can reveal classic pericardial friction rub, due to contact between visceral and parietal layers.

Classic rub consists of three distinctive components linked, respectively, to ventricular systole, early diastolic filling and atrial contraction, and it's loudest if heard at lower left stern border [64].

Electrocardiogram present diffuse ST segment elevation in all leads except aVr and often V1. PR segment depression is another common finding in acute pericarditis, always standing alone without ST elevation [66].

Modest elevations of white blood cells and aspecific elevation of cardiac ezymes (total CPK and MB fraction, Troponin I) are often observed [67].

Chest radiography is usually normal in uncomplicated forms of acute idiopathic pericarditis with small pulmonary infiltrates in mycoplasma infections. Bacterial pericarditis is often associated with radiologic picture of severe pneumonia [62].

Pulmonary vascular congestion may reveal presence of severe myocarditis, while tubercolosis has typical radiologic picture.

Echocardiography is normal in patient without pericardial effusion; moderate or severe effusions may suggest an alternative diagnosis to acute pericarditis [63].

There are no established guidelines for management of acute pericarditis; initial management have to be focused on primary disease.

Acute idiopathic pericarditis is self – limited without complications in about 70 – 90% of patients. If laboratory tests support diagnosis, symptomatic treatment with nonsteroidal anti-inflammatory drugs (NSAIDs) should be started.

Ibuprofen has to be preferred to indomethacin because of it's better safety profile and it is administered in a range from 600 to 800mg three times daily for two weeks.

Patients who respond slowly to NSAIDs may require narcotic analgesics or brief cours of corticosteroid, or both [68].

2.3. Constrictive Pericarditis

Constrictive pericarditis represents end stage of pericardial inflammatory process. Although various clinical conditions can lead to this final stage, in the modern world etiology is most commonly infectious, postsurgical or by radiation injury (Table 5). Usually constrictive process follows primum movens by little or several months but it takes many years to reach final result of dense fibrosis, often associated with calcification and adhesions of parietal and visceral pericardium.

Clinical onset is dominated by signs and symptoms of right heart failure [62].

Pathophysiological consequence of clinical process is characterized by restricted filling of all cardiac chambers with elevation of filling pressures in all chambers and systemic and pulmonary veins.

Early diastolic phase is characterized by abnormally rapid ventricles filling following elevated atrial pressures and accentuated early diastolic ventricular suction.

When intracardiac volumes reaches higher limit and pericardium becames not compliant, systemic vein congestion occurs and hepatic congestion, peripheral edema and ascites ('till anasarca) can be evident.

Reduced cardiac index is a consequence of impaired filling while myocardial contractile function is preserved, but ejection fraction can be reduced because of reduced preload [69].

Common clinical presentation, as previously mentioned, is those of right – sided heart failure with normal ventricular systolic function at echocardiographic evaluation.

Table 5. Causes of constrictive pericarditis

IDIOPATHIC
AUTOIMMUNE DISORDERS
IRRADIATION
UREMIA
POSTSURGICAL
POST - TRAUMATIC
INFECTIOUS
METHYSERGIDE THERAPY
NEOPLASTIC
IMPLANTABLE DEVICES

At early stages patient presents with lower limbs edema and some degree of hepatic congestion.

As disease goes on, hepatic congestion can progress to jaundice, ascites until anasarca and cardiac cirrhosis together with exertional dyspnea, cough and orthopnea linked to elevated pulmonary venous pressures [62].

At physical examination marked elevation of jugular venous pressure is clearly evident, and "pericardial knock" is audible as an early diastolic sound best heard at the left sterna border of cardiac apex: it is slightly earlier with an higher acoustic frequency than a third heart sound. Pericardial knock correspond to early cessation of ventricular filling.

Abdominal examination reveals hepatomegaly, with or without ascites and jaundice. Lower limbs edema is usually present [62].

There is not a specific electrocardiographic pattern with non specific T waves abnormalities and signs of left atrial abnormalities.

Chest radiography shows right atrial enlargement, while pericardial calcification is seen in small percentage of patients.

M and B- mode echocardiogram reveals pericardial thickening and displacement of interventricular septum during early diastole, dilation of hepatic veins with distention of inferior vena cava with breathing [63].

For whom to concern management of constrictive pericarditis, this is a progressive disease and surgical pericardiectomy is the only radical treatment [70].

Medical therapy is based upon diuretics employment and salt restriction to obtain symptomatic relief of fluid overload and peripheral edema.

Beta – blockers and calcium antagonists should be avoided, while digoxin is recommended as initial treatment in patients with atrial fibrillation [70].

Ischemic Heart Disease and Chronic Kidney Disease

1. Introduction

Patients with chronic kidney disease (CKD), especially in those with end stage renal disease (ESRD), show reduced life expectance [71]. Falling in glomerular filtration rate (eGFR) represent a powerful graded predictor of cardiovascular morbidity, mortality and all-causes of mortality. Even subclinical renal dysfunction such as microalbuminuria, increase cardiovascular risk. Thus, ESRD patients express higher risk for premature death, due largely to cardiovascular causes. CKD alone is an independent risk factor for presence, development and severity of coronary artery disease (CAD). Risks for adverse effect on prognosis from cardiovascular disease associated with CKD includes increased mortality after an acute coronary syndrome and after percutaneous coronary intervention (PCI) with or without stenting. Furthermore, CKD patients are more likely to present with atypical symptoms, which may delay diagnosis and adversely affecting cardiovascular outcomes.

However, patients with eGFR below 60 mL/min per 1.73 m2 have more probability to die than develop ESRD. Medicare beneficiaries with kidney disease who are not yet on dialysis are 60% more likely to have a billing claim submitted for the diagnosis of cardiovascular disease (CVD), and 70% more likely to have a claim submitted for "atherosclerotic heart disease". At the time starting dialysis therapy, majority of patients had established CAD. In diabetic renal transplant candidates, 30% will have one or more lesion with greater than 75% stenosis. ESRD patients have more numerous and severe coronary artery lesions and more severe myocardial dysfunction when compared to patients who undergo evaluation for CAD without CKD.

Prevalence of angiographically significant CAD ranges from 25% in young, nondiabetic hemodialysis patients to about 85% in older ESRD patients with longstanding diabetes [72]. Thus, risk of cardiac death in dialysis patients younger than age 45 is 100 times greater than that the general population.

It has been estimated that in-hospital mortality rates in patients with acute myocardial infarction (AMI) increases within the degree of renal impairment: 2% in patients with normal renal function, 6% in those with mild renal dysfunction, 14% in those with moderate renal dysfunction, 21% in those with severe renal dysfunction, and 30% in those with ESRD. Similarly, a comparable directional trend has been observed for increasing risk of postdischarge death with advancing degrees of CKD. In patients on long-term dialysis who were hospitalized for a first myocardial infarct, the mortality rate from cardiac causes was 40.8% at 1 year, 51.8% at 2 years, and 70.2% at 5 years.

In this way, more effective strategy to reduce cardiovascular morbidity and mortality in this population would be to stratify patients with mild renal impairment to prevent and treat more severe and advances forms of CKD [73].

CKD is classified in 5 stages and detectable risk for procedural complications typically occurs with an eGFR below of 60 mL/min/1.73m2. This topic review will focus on advanced stage of CKD, which is often composed of patients with ESRD on maintenance dialysis.

2. Risk Factor for Coronary Artery Disease in Chronic Kidney Disease Patients

In patients with CKD, risk factors for CAD could be classify as either "traditional" or "nontraditional" [74] (see table I on Epidemiology).

Given the large number of traditional and nontraditional uremia-related factors that have been shown to be associated with increased cardiovascular risk and mortality in CKD, nephrologists do not yet know which risk factors should be used for screening in clinical practice. Since the role and description of several cardiovascular risk factors have been the topic of extensive reviews in both the non - renal and renal literature, in this chapter number of risk factors to be described has been limited only to those with greater importance for the cardiovascular stratification [75].

Traditional risk factors are those of Framingham Heart Study that have been used to estimate the risk of developing symptomatic ischemic heart disease. Most of the traditional CAD risk factors, such as older age, diabetes mellitus, systolic hypertension, LVH, and low high-density lipoprotein (HDL) cholesterol, are highly prevalent in patients with CKD.

In this patients, the cardiovascular risk conferred by many traditional risk factors, such as diabetes, older age, and LVH, shows a strong parallelism in comparison to that described in the general population.

However, some controversy have been suggested about the effectiveness of the Framingham risk equation to assessment the degree of CAD risk in subjects with CKD. Two different interpretation have been proposed in this regard. First, other factors (nontraditional risk factors) that are not included in Framingham risk equations may play an important role in promoting ischemic heart disease in subjects with CKD. Second, traditional risk factors may have a qualitatively and quantitatively different risk relationship with CVD in CKD compared with the general population. Indeed, usually CKD patients have more severe exposure to hypertension than subjects without CKD.

Several non – traditional risk factors, such as hyperhomocysteinemia, oxidant stress, dyslipidemia, and elevated inflammatory markers, are associated with atherosclerosis. In addition, oxidant stress and inflammation have been proposed as the primary mediators explaining burden of CAD in CKD. Other risk factors, such as anemia, are associated with cardiomyopathy, whereas abnormal calcium and phosphorus metabolism is associated with vascular remodeling and calcifications, developing in noncompliant vessels. Anemia is considered major risk factor for development of left ventricular hypertrophy (LVH) and left ventricular dilatation. Although partial anemia correction with erythropoietic-stimulating agents (ESA) induces LVH regression, current information does not suggest any cardiovascular outcome benefit of normalized haemoglobin levels in CKD patients.

Secondary hyperparathyroidism (sHPT) and alterations in calcium and phosphorus metabolism, starting earlier in stage 3 and 4 CKD, may accelerate calcifying and atherosclerosis allowing coronary artery disease.

All these putative risk factors can be associated with increased risk for either all-cause mortality or CVD in various stages of CKD.

After stratification for age, cardiovascular mortality remains ≈5-fold higher in dialysis patients than in general population, even at the extremes of age. This phenomena is likely due to both a high case fatality rate and a high prevalence of CAD.

A mortality rate has been observed after acute myocardial infarction both in dialysis patients and in patients with heart failure. In dialysis patients, mortality after 1 and 2 years from myocardial infarction has been estimated approximately in 59% and 73%, respectively, which is much higher than after acute myocardial infarction in general population, even in those subjects with comorbid conditions such as diabetes, atherosclerosis or peripheral vascular disease. In the Worcester Heart Attack Study, approximately 75% of diabetic men and two thirds of diabetic women discharged after an acute myocardial infarction were still alive 2 years later. Other study have been also confirmed a sensible survival reduction after development of de novo heart failure in dialysis patients than observed in the general population. The prevalence of atherosclerosis, heart failure, and LVH remains extremely high in dialysis patients. In ESRD starting dialysis therapy, prevalence of CAD is approximately 40% and LVH is already present in most of them.

3. Cardiovascular Assessment of the Renal Transplant Candidate

In patient with ESRD who is eligible for renal transplantation, atherosclerotic CAD, whether symptomatic or asymptomatic, is associated with an increased incidence of allograft failure and mortality. Based on this data, transplant candidates with angina or evidence of previous myocardial infarction typically undergo coronary angiography as a part of their pre -

transplant evaluation, and subsequent transplantation may be denied if CAD is extensive and not amenable to re - vascularization.

Both National Kidney Foundation [73] and American Heart Association Task Forces [76] have recently recommended that patients with ESRD must be considered in the highest risk group for cardiovascular events. Since coronary revascularization may improve prognosis in dialysis patients, precocious identification of patients at risk for cardiac events could induce changes in clinical management in the attempt to prevent fatal complications [77,78]. Unluckly, symptoms of CAD may be unclear or absent in dialysis patients [79], diagnosis of CAD may be mystified.

KDOQI clinical practice guidelines for CAD in dialysis patients recommended a baseline electrocardiogram at dialysis initiation and at yearly intervals. CKD patients with increase QRS length have approximately 15% greater risk incident of chronic heart disease and 13% greater risk of incidence of CAD. Prolongation of QT interval have been also found independently associated with adverse outcomes [73].

Coronary angiography is the gold standard in CAD identification and should be considered in stable ESRD patients with evidence for inducible myocardial ischemia, unstable patients with acute coronary syndrome (performed urgently for ST-segment elevation myocardial infarction) and in those patients with a left ventricular ejection fraction below 40% [80]. However, cost and complications make the indication of invasive cardiac procedures in ESRD patients as screening test for CAD debatable. This is why scientific societies and international guidelines strongly suggest the extensive use of non-invasive strategies for detecting CAD in ESRD patients. In addition, coronary angiography does not provide functional information.

Routine echocardiogram in all dialysis patients after they achieved "dry weight" targets is strongly recommended by KDOQI guidelines [73]. Moreover, echocardiogram should be performed 1 to 3 months after starting dialysis treatment on an inter - dialytic day for hemodialysis and at 3-year intervals thereafter. Diminished left ventricular systolic function is independently associated with onset of chronic heart failure and ischemic heart disease and it is not accurately detected by anamnesis physical examination or routine test such as chest radiography.

Non - invasive coronary CT angiography may be problematic in dialysis patients because of medial calcification interfering with angiographic interpretation. Another problem is represented by the large bore intravenous lines for rapid injection of radiocontrast media. Non-invasive gadolinium-based magnetic resonance angiography in patients with severe CKD is not longer recommended because of concerns about nephrogenic fibrosing dermopathy. On the other hand, values of imaging without contrast media is unknown.

Exercise testing is hampered by the inability of many patients to attain an adequate workload and studies performed using dipyridamole thallium-201 have shown conflicting results [81].

The diagnostic and prognostic role of dobutamine stress echocardiography in risk stratification has been established in renal transplant candidates [82-86]. However, this diagnostic test is characterized by the elevated incidence of hypertension in ESRD patients and the risk of development ventricular arrhythmias that could represent a contraindication to the use of adrenergic stress in this population [87]. In non uremic patients, Dipyridamole Stress Echocardiography is not limited by hypertension related complications and it has a similar prognostic value as compared to Dobutamine Stress Echocardiography [88]. There are extensive data available in literature demonstrating in cardiac disease patients that prognostic and diagnostic values are similar in both dobutamine and dipyridamole stress tests. In a meta-analysis [89] of twelve studies involving thallium-201 scintigraphy and dobutamine stress echocardiography (DSE), ESRD patients with inducible ischemia had approximately six-times risk of myocardial infarction and four-times the risk of cardiac death as patients without inducible defects.

In asymptomatic subjects from general population the presence of inducible ischemia is estimated up to 4%, three times higher in males compared to females, and the prevalence increases with age [90]. The prevalence reaches 10% when two or more major cardiovascular risk factors are added [91, 92], and up to 15-30% when myocardial infarction is present.

Subjects with ESRD who do not have angina or who have atypical symptoms of CAD pose a difficult management approach because many of them, particularly diabetic patients, present underlying CAD [93].

Few data are available regarding prevalence of CAD in asymptomatic ESRD patients and these have only been performed in diabetic patients. Data from international literature [93, 94] show how approximately 41% of asymptomatic diabetic patients with ESRD awaiting transplantation had significant CAD.

In recent study [95] prevalence of silent CAD in asymptomatic ESRD patients result in more than two times higher than in the general population. In fact, using dipyridamole stress tests, CAD have been detected in almost 10% of asymptomatic dialysis patients. However, in our population timely CAD diagnosis does not seem to improve the prognosis in terms of total and cardiovascular mortality. In presence of CKD it would be opportune to look for a silent CAD before than patients start HD therapy.

4. Biomarkers for Coronary Artery Disease in Chronic Kidney Disease

CKD is a complex condition, where kidney function decline is accompanied by several metabolic changes affecting almost all organ systems. Biomarkers have been associated with adverse outcomes. These biomarkers are different in patients with CKD compared to the general population in the prediction of morbidity and mortality. The use of the biomarkers should serve to stratify the patient at high risk of cardiovascular (Figure 5).

The use of high-sensitivity C-reactive protein (HS-CRP) has extensively been proposed for risk assessment by reflecting chronic inflammation in CKD patients at intermediate risk of CAD [96]. HS-CRP has recently emerged as a useful biomarker for vascular inflammation associated with atherosclerosis and determination of HS-CRP levels is currently recommended by the American Heart Association in all patients at a risk of CAD. Its levels can be used for estimating the development and severity of atherosclerosis both in general population and in CKD patients with or without cardiovascular manifestations.

Natriuretic peptides such as brain natriuretic peptide (BNP) and N-terminal pro-BNP (NT-proBNP) are commonly used in the diagnosis and evaluation of heart failure [97]. However, their utility in patients with CKD is less clear as renal dysfunction itself can be associated with elevated concentrations of these biomarkers. Given high prevalence of LVH, left ventricular systolic dysfunction and CAD in patients with CKD, diagnosis or exclusion of heart failure becomes important in this population.

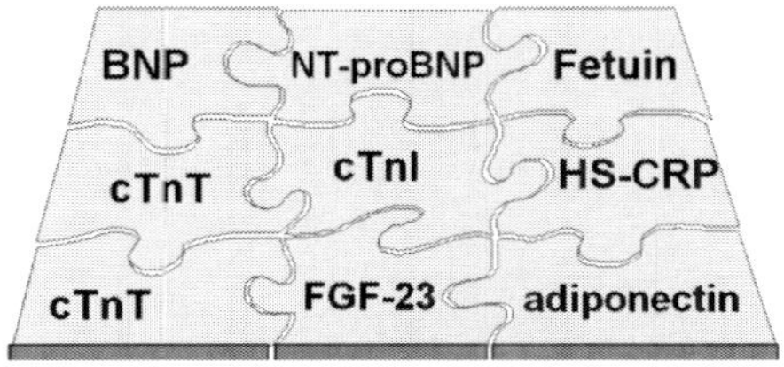

Figure 5. The complicated puzzle of traditional and emerging biomarkers for screening cardiovascular risk in chronic kidney disease.

BNP reflect cardiac filling pressure not limited to the left side of the heart. In acute coronary syndrome, BNP/NT-proBNP has been reported to be an extremely powerful prognostic indicator and recently, BNP/NT-proBNP has also been shown to be useful in stable CAD patients. Circulating BNP levels have been correlated with disease severity as assessed by number of stenotic coronary arteries and CAD prognostic index in chronic dialysis patients with CAD, suggesting utility in diagnosis and follow-up of stable CAD in dialysis patients.

Cardiac troponins (cTn), has been proposed as another traditional biomarker in cardiac evaluation of CKD patients [98]. The kidneys participate in clearance of cTnT but its serum levels, even in dialysis patients, appears referring to cardiac synthesis. While a dynamic rise and fall in cTn with appropriate clinical signs or symptoms is suggestive of acute coronary syndromes, persistent elevations in cTn may reflect other forms of cardiac injury such as strain from hypertension, volume overload, especially in dialysis patients, or LVH. Consistent associations of elevated levels of cTnT isoforms with all-cause and cardiac death risk in asymptomatic CKD patients have been found; a recent meta-analysis has clearly shown that cTnT >0.10 ng/ml was associated with more than doubling of the mortality experienced by patients with lower cTnT levels.

The most cost-effective combination of biomarkers for risk stratification in dialysis patients might be cTnT and HS-CRP, but this sentebce is controversial. In asymptomatic non-dialysis depend CKD patients, circulating cTnT and cTnI have been found elevated in at least a third of patients, but only cTnT has been predictive of death. Risk in relation to cTnI has been more heterogeneous, and may reflect lack of assay standardization and/or use of a broader range of cut-points.

On the basis of these data, the U.S. Food and Drug Administration approved the measurement of cTnT in dialysis patients for the indication of risk stratification and mortality prediction, however, utility of this information in clinical practice remains unclear.

New emerging biomarkers are quickly becoming popular in the stratification of CKD patient at risk for CAD.

An important systemic extraosseus mineralization inhibitor thus far identified is fetuin-A or a2-HS-glycoprotein [99]. Fetuin-A is mainly produced in the liver and inhibits de novo formation and precipitation of basic calcium phosphate. Consequentially, this biomarker can inhibit calcification in circulation without affecting the normal bone mineralization. In patients with ESRD serum fetuin-A levels are significantly reduced. Low levels of fetuin-A are related to increased cardiovascular mortality and fetuin-A levels inversely correlate with the extent and grade of coronary calcification in dialysis patients.

High levels of the phosphaturic hormone fibroblast growth factor 23 (FGF-23) have been associated with cardiovascular events both in non-dialysis depend CKD and in hemodialysis patients [100]. This data suggest that FGF-23 might be able to predict cardiovascular mortality in each degree of CKD.

Higher serum level of adiponectin have been associated with a lower cardiovascular risk in patients with CKD, suggesting that a high serum adiponectin acts as a protective factor for cardiovascular system [101]. In contrast, some studies have shown that a high serum level of adiponectin is associated with an increase of CVD events or high mortality in patients with congestive heart failure, overt CAD, or type 2 diabetes. Thus, the significance of adiponectin as an indicator of prognosis seems to be still controversial and the mechanisms responsible for these apparently contradictory findings remain unclear.

5. Therapy of Coronary Artery Disease in Chronic Kidney Disease

5.1. Optimal Medical Therapy

Patient with incipient CKD should be considered to be at highest cardiovascular risk, with an expected rate of CAD death that is many-fold the rate expected for a patient without CKD. Thus, CKD is more than a cardiovascular risk equivalent. Hence, in CKD patients, therapeutic strategies should be undertaken that are even more aggressive than those recommended in conventional guidelines.

It is clearly imperative to strongly to promote smoking cessation at any CKD stage. Lifestyle changes, including balance diets, low salt and phosphate diet, weight reduction to a target body mass index <25 kg/m2, limitation of alcohol intake and exercise for 60 minutes per day most days of the week, could be reduce cardiovascular morbidity.

Hypertension is the most prevalent risk factor for both CKD and CAD. Renal dysfunction and hypertension are inextricably linked. Current guidelines from U.S. National Kidney Foundation and the seventh report of the Joint National Committee on Prevention, Detection, Evaluation, and Treatment of High Blood Pressure recommend a target blood pressure below 130/80 mmHg for prevention of cardiovascular events and progression of kidney disease in patients with a GFR below 60 mL/min for more than 3 months [32].

Despite multiple medications employment, most published series on CKD patients indicate that nearly 80% of this patients have hypertension, and that it is adequately controlled in only 30% [102]. Drugs interfering with renin-angiotensin aldosterone system (RAAS), such as an angiotensin-converting enzyme inhibitor (ACEI) or an angiotensin receptor blocker (ARB) are first choice therapy. Several clinical outcomes evidence for the benefit of ACEI/ARB in the general population are also extends to CKD patients. Unfortunately, treatment with ACEI/ARB may result in worsening hyperkalemia in patients with ESRD. As tolerated, the clinician should consider adjusting the dialytic regimen to optimize potassium balance and continue treatment with ACEI/ARB. To date, available evidence indicates that patients with ESRD appear to benefit from ACEI/ARB therapy provided the serum potassium and blood pressure can be adequately controlled.

Using an ACEI/ARB as first – line therapy, antihypertensive regimen can be further modified according to blood pressure lowering efficacy and CAD event reduction.

Beta-blockers can be used as both an antihypertensive and an anti-ischemic agent. In patients with both CKD and heart failure, beta-blockers can contribute with improvement of left ventricular ejection fraction and reducing rates of hospitalization, sudden death, and all-cause mortality. Large relative risk reductions in all-cause mortality have demonstrated in patients with CKD who receive beta-blockers therapy after CAD events [102 - 104].

When arterial blood pressure cannot be adequately controlled with ACEI/ARB and beta-blockers therapy, additional antihypertensive agents can be added to bring to the target pressure values.

To reach the optimal blood pressure targets proposed in guidelines for non-CKD patients may be difficult in patients with incipient CKD and ESRD [104].

Patients with ESRD who depend on hemodialysis do not benefit from aggressive blood pressure control. In this population, aggressive lowering of blood pressure results in increased mortality. Hypotension may be associated with malnutrition, which is common in dialysis patients. In addition, hypotension predicts a poor prognosis in heart failure, which commonly affects many hemodialysis patients [105]. Given the high rates of severe CAD in ESRD, hypotension during dialysis could be related to clinical and subclinical myocardial ischemia, which should be suspected in the presence of chest discomfort, shortness of breath, ST-segment depression on electrocardiography, or elevations of cardiac biomarkers on blood testing.

Lipid metabolism is disturbed in CKD, with gradual shift to the uremic lipid profile as kidney function deteriorates, which is further deteriorated by the presence of comorbidities such as diabetes and obesity [106]. Apart from quantitative differences, major qualitative changes in lipoproteins can be observed, such as oxidization and modification to small and dense low-density lipoprotein (LDL), which render the particles more atherogenic.

It has been noted that these abnormalities contribute to the development of CV events, and they may lead to the progression of CKD. Lipid-lowering treatment with statins in CKD patients using statins induce an important benefit on cardiovascular outcomes and, perhaps, with more controversial evidence, on the progression of kidney disease. Available evidences suggest that lipid-lowering therapy confer similar benefits both in patients with CKD and ESRD [107]. The safety profile of lipid- lowering therapy with statins in CKD is indistinguishable from that observed in people with normal renal function. Consequently, lipid- lowering therapy with statins should be part of the standard treatment of patients with CKD with and without CAD.

In CKD patients with diabetes, blood glucose control to a target glycohemoglobin <7 mg/dL can be expected to reduce rates of microvascular disease such as retinopathy and, to a lesser extent, clinically important atherosclerotic disease elsewhere (such as myocardial infarction, stroke, cardiovascular death [108].

Low-dose aspirin [81 mg daily) has been associated with a 20% to 30% reduction in the risk of stroke, AMI, and CVD death across many populations [109]. The effect of aspirin on renal end points is unknown; however, given its cardiovascular protective effect, it is recommended for adult patients with ESRD. For those who are aspirin intolerant, general cardiology guidelines recommend the use of clopidogrel, although there are no published studies of clopidogrel on cardiovascular outcomes in the setting of ESRD.

5.2. Revascularization Options in Non-Hemodialysis-Dependent Chronic Kidney Disease Patients

The relative protection conferred by revascularization in patients with CKD or ESRD and established CAD is remains still unknown. Although observational studies have suggested that revascularization procedures may improve survival when compared with patients under medical therapy alone, there are some limitation that should be considered. One of the most important is given by the bias of selection of the "healthiest" patients for higher-risk treatment alternatives. Patients with mild renal dysfunction are generally treated with revascularization while those with more severe degrees of CKD and greatest risk of subsequent events undergo might be treated more conservatively.

5.3. Coronary Artery Bypass Grafting

In CKD patients who do not require dialysis therapy preoperative GFR (usually estimated using the Cockroft-Gault method) is a better indicator of early death after coronary artery bypass grafting (CABG) than is serum creatinine, in term of postoperative adverse outcome, predominantly acute renal failure [110,111]. Patients with less than 30 mL/min/1.73 m2, in whom the probability to experience postoperative acute renal failure is about 20 times greater than patients with normal renal function, use of internal mammary artery grafts using in CKD patients seems to be the protective compared with the use of venous grafts [112].

Survival rates after CABG in no dialysis-dependent CKD patients are consistently lower than in the general population with normal renal function. However, lack of homogeneity and standardization of these studies makes it difficult to interpret.

In contrast to patients with normal or mild impaired renal function, those with ESRD have patients 3-fold greater mortality ranges and about 2-fold the complications of surgery, including mediastinitis, stroke and need for prolonged mechanical ventilation [112]. These condition concomitantly with others comorbidities, such as decreased left ventricular ejection fraction, chronic obstructive pulmonary disease, severe distal disease and generalized atherosclerosis increase morbidity rates and delay intensive care unit and hospitalization.

It has been estimated that survival rate after routine CABG in ESRD patients ranges from 71% to 95% at 1 year, 44% to 84% at 3 year and 32% to 82% at 5 year. Variables associated with death are similar to those for patients without ESRD.

In patients with both ESRD and diabetes, the 5-year survival rate after revascularization procedures is substantially lower than that in patients with ESRD alone.

5.4. Percutaneous Intervention

In patients undergoing percutaneous coronary intervention (PCI) mortality rates is significantly higher in patients with creatinine clearances less than 30 mL/min than in patients with normal or mild impaired renal function. In addition, patients with GFR less than 30 mL/min present higher rate of acute renal failure both due to the risk of contrast-induced nephropathy and to the risk of developing atheroembolic renal failure compared with the other group [113,114].

One year mortality after PCI increases from 1.1% when the GFR is greater than 75 mL/min to 2.9% when the GFR is less than 60 mL/min [115] and in this period composite endpoint of death and myocardial infarction is higher in CKD patients than in non-CKD ones [116].

In ESRD patients with more comorbid conditions and more severe vascular calcification, the likelihood of failure after PCI is higher than in patients with normal or mild impaired renale function.

Several retrospective studies indicate that ESRD and non-ESRD populations have similar initial rates of angiographic and periprocedural myocardial infarction after PCI procedures showing similar rates of restenosis [113,114].

Data show that one year after the index procedure, the mortality rate is almost 3-fold higher in ESRD patients than in non-ESRD patients [113,115].

Drug-eluting stents have substantially reduced restenosis and frequency of repeating procedures after stent placement. ESRD patients undergoing placement of drug-eluting stents present similar target-vessel revascularization than non-ESRD patients. This reasonable risk of restenosis was offset by increased death in the ESRD group, which might mask the true risk of clinically significant restenosis [117].

5.5. Comparison of Revascularization Techniques

CABG provided a survival benefit in comparison with PCI. However, in a group of patients with GFR upper than 60 mL/min, this beneficial effect disappears [118]. This information could be interpreted that patients with GFR of more than 60 mL/min may be considered part of the general, unaffected population.

Rate of restenosis seems to be higher with PCI than with CABG in CKD patients. In fact, patients with GFR lower than 60 mL/min who underwent stent placement show 3 times more probability to repeat intervention likely than patients who underwent CABG [119, 120].

Drug-eluting stent was associated with a reduced risk of target-lesion revascularization and angiographic restenosis at 1 year, compared with bare-metal stents in CKD patients [121].

Unluckly, there are no available studies that compare drug-eluting stents and surgical revascularization as a means of coronary revascularization in CKD patients.

Long-term survival rates are higher in ESRD patients who undergo CABG than in those who undergo PTCA [118,122,123]. Evidence from USRDS national database show that ESRD patients undergoing CABG have significantly higher long-term survival rates at 2 and 5 years than those patients who underwent PTCA. In addition, reduction of both all-cause death and cardiac death, have been observed in patient treated with surgical procedures [122,123].

Drug-eluting stents, are associated with significant reductions in target-vessel revascularization, all-causes of death, myocardial infarction and target-vessel revascularization, compared with bare-metal stents in ESRD patients [124].

Coronary artery bypass grafting show better long-term survival, but higher in-hospital death. However, PCI using drug-eluting stents may represent a valid alternative in patients in whom multiple comorbid conditions preclude surgery.

Anemia and Chronic Kidney Disease

1. Introduction

Anemia is the most common complication of patient with chronic kidney disease (CKD). By definition, anemia is the state with a hemoglobin (Hb) level <11.5 g/dL in women and <13.5 g/dL in adult men (in ederly men <12.5 g/dL) [125].

Anemia in CKD is characterized by normocytic and normochromic red blood cells (RBCs), an inappropriately low reticolocyte count for the degree of anemia, and a hypoplastic erytroid bone marrow, with normal leukopoiesis and megakaryocytopoiesis. Anemia is a constant feature of chronic renal failure and hemoglobin typically declines in parallel with falling in glomerular filtration rate (GFR). Development of anemia is often complicated by co-morbidities, such as diabetes, hypertension, severe heart failure, neoplasia or chronic inflammation.

Anemia in chronic renal failure begins early in development of kidney disease and in some patients is clinically evident by stage 3 or an estimated GFR of less than 60 mL/min. With progressive destruction of kidney tissue and consequently the loss of kidney function, the degree of anemia increases, typically progressing in parallel with the deterioration of renal function.

Males have 30% greater risk of developing anemia as compared to their female counterparts. Although males have higher hemoglobin values, they also have higher rates of advanced CKD. There has been a lower prevalence of anemia in current smokers, which has been attributed to secondary erythrocytosis.

Data from Obrador [126] et al showed that among predialysis patients, 68% of those with advanced CKD who required renal replacement therapy had a hematocrit less than 30 mg/dL; among these, 51% of patients had a hematocrit less than 28 mg/dL. Furthermore, although anemia is not as common in earlier stages of chronic kidney disease, patients with stage 3 disease have a prevalence of concurrent anemia of 5.2%, whereas those with stage 4 disease have a prevalence of concurrent anemia of 44.1%. In this context, approximately 30% of patients with anemia are treated prior to reaching advanced stages of CKD [127].

Anemia is common in elderly people [128]. There is a greater prevalence of anemia of CKD in those older than 60 years, as compared to those aged between 46 and 60 years. This is probably due to the greater rate of CKD in older individuals, as well as the lower estimated GFR that are associated with aging.

Racial disparities in hemoglobin (Hb) levels among both adults and children with CKD are well established [129]. Black adults typically initiate dialysis with significantly lower Hb compared to whites, and African-American race has been shown to be a significant risk factor for anemia among children and teenagers on dialysis. Among adults with earlier stages of non-dialysis CKD, anemia is more prevalent in African-American compared to white patients.

Morbidity and mortality depend greatly on the underlying etiology of the patient's anemia as well as the stage of the disease, whether early or advanced. In fact, in individuals with advanced stages of CKD, etiology of anemia tends to be multifactorial (i.e. decreased RBC production due to lack of erythropoietin, increased RBC destruction due to hemolysis, as well as increased blood loss due to multiple venipunctures for an array of indications) [130].

2. Causes of Anemia in Chronic Kidney Disease

Anemia associated with CKD is primarily due to failure of kidney endocrine function, resulting in deficient levels of renal erhytropoietin (EPO) production.

Many pathophysiologic mechanisms leading to anemia in CKD have been clarified by clinical and experimental observations such as the effect of dialysis treatment in chronic uremia and therapy with human recombinant EPO (rHuEPO). The driving force for renal EPO production is extrarenal tissue hypoxia, which results from an imbalance between delivery and metabolic needs [128].

In early CKD, the dominant mechanism of anemia is suppression of red blood cells (RBCs) syntesis by uremic toxins and from shortened RBCs survival [131]. As CKD advances, EPO production decreases and EPO levels become lower than those expected for the degree of anemia. Significant EPO deficiency exist as the biofeedback mechanism becomes progressively impaired.

In progressive CKD, the degree of anemia is in general proportional to the severity of azotemia. Correlation of hematocrit (Htc) with GFR, blood urea nitrogen (BUM) or serum creatinine is imprecise among patients. However, as renal function approaches 20% of normal, majority of patients become anemic with Ht levels less than 30%. Average EPO levels of 20-25 mU/mL in anemic CKD patients are above abnormal values in non - uremic individuals only reaching 25% the level of EPO production expected for the degree of anemia [132]. Thus, main feature in anemia of CKD patients is inadequate production of EPO by the diseased kidney in toto.

Although involved kidney continues to produce relatively low levels of EPO, it is incapable of augmenting EPO production adequately in response to an appropriate anemic hypoxic stimulus. Maintenance of appropriate plasma levels of EPO during severe anemia would require that residual renal tissue have the capacity to increase EPO synthesis by about 5 to 20 fold. It have been shown that in normal kidney responds to hypoxia or anemia by recruitment of additional production sites isolated in the peritubular or vascular space. In injured kidney, this site are impaired leading to charges in hemoglobin-oxygen affinity of uremic erythrocytes.

Nephropaties lead the kidney incapable to provide an adequate and chronic EPO production in response to anemic hypoxic stimulus. The bilateral nephrectomized patients shown an absolute deficiency of endogenous EPO production and invariably develops much lower levels of Hct. An exception to the rule is given by autosomal dominant polycystic kidney disease, which is typically associated with higher EPO levels and mild to non anemia.

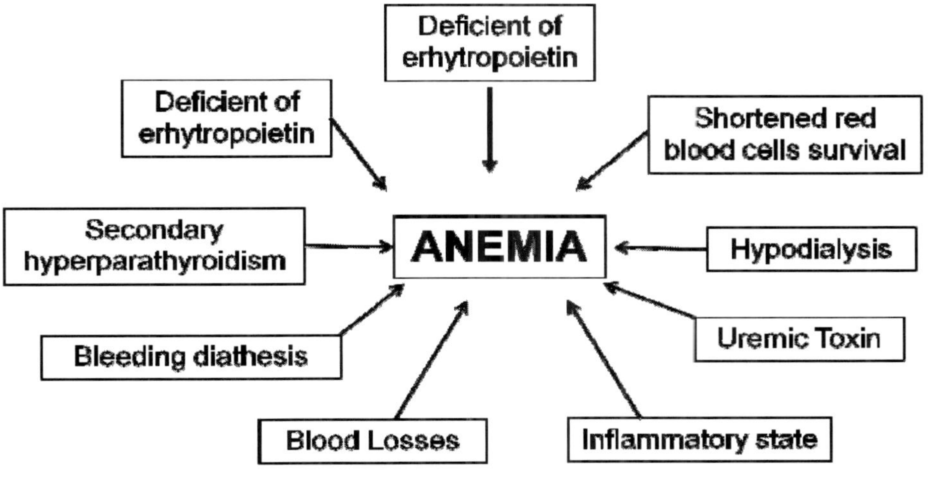

Figure 6. Anemia etiology in chronic kidney disease.

3. Other Anemia Causes

Although inadequate EPO production is the principal factor in the pathogenesis of anemia in CKD; other factors contributes to cause the mild anemia that persists despite the use of therapeutic erythropoiesis-stimulating agents (ESA) (see figure 6). Most important among these are shortened erythrocyte survival, blood loss, iron and other nutritional deficiencies, and perhaps the effects of uremic inhibitor on the stimulatory action of EPO and the bone marrow [131].

Erythrocyte survival is shortened in chronic renal failure, decreasing from normal 100-140 days to hardly 70-80 days. Both mechanic and metabolic factors may explain the decreased survival of RBCs. In hemodialysis patients repeated vascular access punctures, residual blood left in dialyzers and bloodlines, occasional blood leaks and blood retention in clotted dialyzers all contribute to ongoing blood loss, resulting on premature removal of circulating erythrocytes. Other important mechanical factor related to hemodialysis include maloclussion of the roller pump, shearing effects from negative pressure in needles and sub-lethal thermal injury. However, modern conductivity sensor have virtually eliminated osmotic injury to the BRCs from hypotonic dialysate.

Metabolic effect of uremic environment include abnormal cation transport across erythrocytes which alters membrane shape, deformability and rigidity favor hemolysis and consequently shortens erythrocyte survival. Hemolysis has been attribuited to either uremic impairment of enzymatic activity or decrease synthesis of membrane cation transport pumps units by uremic reticulocytes.

Because uremic RBCs survive normally when transfused into healthy recipients and normal RBCs have a reduced lifespan in uremic patients, retention of one or more uremic solutes in the plasma is believed to be responsible for the hemolysis. In addition, it has been seen that starting of dialytic treatment can improve anaemia and the and intensive dialysis treatment is able to normalized erythrocytes survival. This data strongly support that erythropoiesis is influenced by the retention of uremic toxins [135].

Secondary hyperparathyroidism (sHPT) can lead to myelofibrosis in CKD patients, and affected patients often require high doses of ESA to achieve target Hb levels [136]. Correction of sHPT either by pharmacologic control or after parathyreidectomy has been shown to reduce ESA requirements needs to reach adequate hematopoietic response in same CKD patients. The improvement of anemia demonstrated following sHPT correction is due to the removal of erytropoietic inhibition.

Uremia has been recognized as an inflammatory state, so the shortened RBCs lifespan may also result from the hemolysis related to inflammation [137]. C-reactive protein levels, a know marker for inflammation, are elevated in pre-dialysis an more so in dialysis patients. Inflammatory cytokines can also inhibit erythropoiesis. Impaired clearance of cytokines, accumulation of advanced glycation end-products (AGEs), atherosclerosis itself and other inflammatory diseases and unrecognized persistent infections have been all implicated. Even if available data are not univocal, Interleukin 1 and 6, tumor necrosis factor- alpha (TNF- α) and interferon- gamma (IFN- α) have been found to antagonize erythropoietin effect on bone marrow proliferation [137]. In this context, TNF- α) has been suggested as a significant individual predictor of ESA requirements in hemodialisis patients. Dialysis procedure *per se* has been linked to increased inflammation [138]. Cytokines levels were directly related to

ESA consumption in haemodialysis patients with significantly higher titles in patients treated with less compatible membranes [139,146].

Premature removal of erythrocytes by the reticuloendothelial system may also occur specially in long-term hemodialysis patients who develop splenomegaly. Splenectomy should be reserved for those patients with either coexistent neutropenia or thrombocytopenia or anemia resistant to ESA.

Many pathological processes can produce iatrogenic hemolysis. Drugs having strong oxidizing potential such as primaquine, quinidine, sulfones and nitrofurantoin, can induce hemolysis by decreasing activity of the hexose monophosphate shunt. Hemolysis can also result from contamination of dialysate by chloramines from city tap-water source, copper, zinc, aluminum and nitrates. Fortunately these cases are mostly of historical interest.

Mild or severe iron deficiency is the most common nutritional factor and is a major impediment to cost-effective use of ESA. Patients with CKD or on maintenance dialysis is prone to anorexia, intercurrent illness and dietary restrictions. Three factors have been implicated in the pathogenesis of iron deficiency in CKD patients [141,142]. First of all blood loss caused by retained RBCs in dialyzers and bloodlines, second bleeding diathesis caused by uremic state and third gastrointestinal malabsortion of iron. In CKD patients iron absortion is impaired by H2 blockers, H+ ion pump inhibitors, nonaluminum-based phosphate binders and aluminum-based phosphate binders [143]. Although iron turnover appears normal in advanced CKD stages, iron utilization is decreased, especially in inflammatory situations [144]. Hepcidin is a recently discovered low-molecular-weight protein that plays an important role in the regulation of iron homeostasis [149]. Hepcidin may be relevant in CKD and explain the often-observed imbalancement in iron metabolism and resistance to ESA. Production of Hepcidin in this patients will depend on iron status, inflammation, anaemia, hypoxia and EPO [146]. In this context it has been proposed that hepcidin could become an important tool to predict ESA responsiveness and to guide treatment with ESA and intravenous iron [150].

Folate deficiency in dialysis patients is uncommon because routine use of supplements during hemodialysis treatment [137,151]. More recently, higher doses of folate have been used to reduce homocysteine levels, although evidence of an associated clinical benefit has yet to be demonstrated.

Carnitine is a metabolic cofactor which is essential for normal fatty acid metabolism [140]. In CKD patients on dialysis have been shown both disordered fatty acid metabolism and a significant deficiency in plasma and tissue carnitine [140]. Decreased levocarine levels are associate with ESA hyporesponsiveness and replacement therapy has improved the response to ESA therapy. Improved RBCs survival and decreased Na/K ATPase activity have benne proposed as potential mechanism [147].

Other pathophysiological factors could interfere with red blood cells turnover in CKD patients. These include malignancy such as myeloma or metastatic cancer, hemolysis induced by systemic diseases as well systemic lupus erytematosus or sickle cell disease, drug-induced anemia and drug-induced bleeding as nonsteroidal anti-inflammatory drus. Infection, inflammation and hypothyroidism all suppress bone marrow erytropoiesis.

4. Anemia Management in Chronic Kidney Disease

Erythropoietin is indispensable for survival, proliferation and differentiation of bone marrow-derived erythroid cells that finally become mature circulating RBCs [138,39]. Most patients with CKD on maintenance dialysis EPO synthesis is insufficient to stimulate adequate levels of erythrocytes production by bone marrow. Although different factors such as iron deficiency, inflammation, infection, uremic toxin other co-morbidity conditions contribute to the development of anemia, a relative deficiency of EPO is the most important factor in this patients [138,139].

Anemia in dialysis patients is associated with increased risk of death from non cardiac and cardiac causes, increased frequency and duration of hospitalization, cardiac dysfunction, reduced quality of life and functional status and reduce exercise tolerance.

Until the advent of EPO therapy, anemia was considered a relatively minor problem for patients suffering from many metabolic consequences of failing kidneys and was managed with transfusions or androgens. Treatment of anemia has assumed more importance given the increasing age of the CKD population. These patients have more frequent and greater degree of ischemic heart and peripheral vascular disease and are increasingly diabetics with both microvascular and macrovascular disease.

4.1. Treatment with Erythropoietic-Stimulating Agents

Clinical trials of rHuEPO alpha were initiated in 1985 to 1986, and replacement therapy with rHuEPO quickly became the most rational therapy for anemia in CKD patients. First treatment reported in hemodialysis patient was in 1987 and approved by the U.S Food and Drug Administration (FDA) in 1989. These initial clinical trials demonstrated that the Ht could be increased by up above 30% in more than 90% of patients, revoluzioning anemia management in both dialysis and non dialysis patients.

Treatment with rHuEPO raised Hb and Htc levels, reduced transfusion requirements and symptoms related to anemia and improved patients' quality of life and functional status. Other subsequent studies have confirmed and extended these initial observations [152].

Epoetin alfa, which must be injected 2 to 3 times per week to achieve efficacy, remained the only exogenous ESA for more than a decade.

At the moment besides epoetin alpha, there are other three available ESA for correcting anemia in patients with CKD: epoetin beta, darbepoetin alfa, and continuous erythropoietin receptor activator (CERA) [153].

Available ESAs can be distinguished by their pharmacokinetic differences (VI). Epoetin alpha and beta has a shorter half-life than darbepoetin alpha and CERA with both intravenous (IV) and subcutaneous (SC) dosing. Subcutaneous administration of epoetin alpha allows for less frequent dosing. Interestingly, the SC effective dose of epoetin alpha is lower than the IV dose despite decreased bioavailability, suggesting that half-life has a greater influence on achieving in vivo effects than speed of absorption. Darbepoetin alpha and CERA that are genetically modified erythropoietin analogue designed for prolonged activity have much longer half-lives, which means they can be administered less frequently. All ESAs are effective in correcting anemia in CKD patients and increasing hemoglobin levels, but the choice of which to use should also take into account their pharmacokinetics and pharmacodynamics, their administration route, and economic issues.

Darbepoietin alpha is a second-generation ESA that is a super-sialylated analogue of EPO, possessing two extra N-linked glycosylation chains. This property confers greater metabolic stability and a lower clearance rate in vivo, and the elimination half-life of this compound in humans after a single intravenous administration is three times greater than epoetin alpha. Darbepoietin can be given less frequently than the standard epoetin, with dosing intervals of once weekly and once every two weeks. In contrast to standard epoetins, dosages requirements for darbepoetin alpha are the same for intravenous and subcutaneous administration. The conversion factor for switching patients from epoetin alpha or beta to darbepoetin alpha is usually quoted as 200:1, but there may be considerable variability in this, depending on the patients population, the dose and the route of administration.

Alternative bioengineering techniques to prolong the half-life of EPO further resulted in development of C.E.R.A., which is a pegylated derivative of epoietin beta with an elimination half-life of around 130 hours when it is administrated either intravenous or subcutaneous.

The expiry of the patents for epoetin alfa and epoetin beta some years ago opened up the way for the production of a number of biosimilars that are now marketed in the European Union. Because biosimilars cannot be identical to their originator, a complex and still-evolving regulatory policy has been generated, but there are still a number of issues concerning international naming, automatic substitution, and safety.

4.2. Initiation and Maintenance Therapy with Erythropoiesis-Stimulating Agents

According to current guidelines, all CKD patients should be investigated and treated if their Hb concentration decreases less than 11 g/dL. Before initiation of ESA therapy, it is essential to exclude and to correct causes of anemia other than EPO deficiency. When ferritin concentration is below 100 mcg/L. Iron supplementation may be administrated [154]. Oral iron supplementation can be considered in patients not yet in dialysis treatment on in peritoneal dialysis, while when the patient is in hemodialysis therapy, iron is best given by intravenous administration. Some patients, especially those not yet in dialysis treatment, may correct their anemia only with iron administration. If ferritin levels is above 100 mcg /L, in the absence of inflammatory or systemic diseases, ESA therapy should be commenced [155]. The usual started dose of epoietin is about 25 to 50 IU/Kg two or three times a week, either by intravenous or by subcutaneous administration. Within 3 to 4 days, an increase in the reticulocytes count it seen, and within 1 to2 weeks, there are a significant rise of Hb concentration. In this way, during the course of 1 month, a significant increase of 1 to 2 g7dL in the Hb correction is usually achieved. ESA dose is increased in stepwise upward titration of 25% to 50% when the patient fail to respond satisfactorily or when there is still an inadequate response. At this point, causes of resistance to EPO therapy should be investigated.

Optimal target of Hb concentration for CKD patients is considered to 11 to 13 g/dL [131], and iron supplementation should be administrated to maximize response to ESA therapy. Starting dose of darbepoietin alpha is usually 20 to 30 mcg once weekly intravenously or subcutaneously, and appropriate starting dose of C.E.R.A. is 30 to 60 mcg every 2 weeks intravenously or subcutaneously.

When Hb concentration remains below 11 g/dL despite increasing doses, hyporesponsiveness to ESA therapy should be considered. There are no absolute definition of hyporesponsiveness to ESA. Major causes of resistance to ESA therapy include iron deficiency, infection and chronic inflammation [144,145]. Poor adherence or reduced compliance must be excluded, especially if patients is self - administering EPO therapy such as peritoneal dialysis or pre - dialysis. Intravenous iron therapy may be useful if there is any doubt about iron deficiency. Folate, vitamin B12 and tyroxine deficiency as well as secondary hyperparathyroidism and aluminum intoxication may be easily excluded [137]. Patients on ACEi and/or AT-II blockers therapy may require higher dose of ESA therapy. Primary bone marrow disorders such as myelodysplastic syndrome, should be investigated by bone marrow investigation if all other causes have been excluded. In suspected antibody-mediated pure red cell aplasia, a bone marrow test may also be necessary.

4.3. Iron Management

Iron is essential for the Hb synthesis and adequate amounts of this mineral are required for the manufacture of new red cells. Under enhanced erythropoietic stimulation, greater amounts of iron are used and many CKD patients, especially hemodialysis patients, have inadequate amounts of available iron to satisfy the increase demands of body marrow. Before initiation of ESA therapy, many CKD patients could have a negative iron balance as a result of poor dietary intake, poor appetite and increase iron looses due to occult and overt blood looses. Looses in hemodialysis patients are up to 5 to 6 mg/day compared with 1 md/day in healthy individuals. This may exceed the absorption capacity of the gastrointestinal tract. Gastrointestinal iron absorption capacity in CKD patients is consistently lower than in healthy individuals especially in the presence of systemic and inflammatory activity. This may by also due to hepcidin upregulation.

Absolute iron deficiency occurs when there are low whole-body iron stores, as indicated by ferritin levels less than 30 mcg /L [155]. Functional iron deficiency occur when there is ample or even increased storage iron but the iron stores fail to release iron rapidly enough to satisfy physiological needs of bone marrow [154]. Despite several markers of iron status are available, none of them is ideal. Serum ferritin is a marker of iron storage but is spuriously raised in inflammatory conditions and liver diseases. Transferrin saturation is a function of the circulating plasma iron in relation to the total iron-binding capacity and is often regarded as a better measure of availale iron, however levels can be highly fluctuant owing to significant diurnal variation in the measurement of plasma iron [155]. Percentage of hypocromic cells and reticulocytes are indirect measurements of iron incorporated into the newly developing or mature red cells. Non one measure of iron status is usually adequate to exclude iron deficiency and the recommended levels for these measures are based on limited scientific evidence. Normal or increased ferritin level and reduced transferring saturation, usually less than 20%, or increased hypocromic red cells less than 10%, suggest functional iron deficiency.

Both European and American guidelines on renal anemia suggest that the ferritin level be maintained in the range of 200 to 500 mcg/L, with an upper limit of 800 mcg /L. Ferritin levels above this threshold do not confer any clinical advantage and may induce iron toxicity. Optimal transferring saturation is above 20 to 30% to ensure available supply of iron to the bone marrow. Percentage of hypocromic red cells levels may be maintained less than 6%.

Iron supplementation is often required in CKD patients [154]. Oral administration is generally poor absorbed in uremics patients and high incidence in gastrointestinal site effect were observed. Intravenous administration of iron has become the standard of care for many CKD patients, particularly those in hemodialysis therapy. In these patients it is easy and practical to give low doses of intravenous iron (e.g., 10 to 20 mg every dialysis session) or alternatively 100 mg weekly. In peritoneal dialysis patients and non dialysis CKD patients such low-dose regimens are impractical and largerdoses may be administrated.

Intravenous iron administration may improve the anemia of CKD in up of 30% of patients not receiving ESA therapy with low ferritin level. In this patients correction of anemia may occur within 2 to 3 weeks after intravenous iron therapy alone. In those patients under ESA therapy intravenous iron administration may enhance the response to the ESA and result in a subsequent reduction of the dose requirements.

Table 6. ESA agents index

Pharmacokinetic Properties of Erythropoiesis-Stimulating Agents			
	IV half-life (h)	SC half-life (h)	Mean (±SEM) CL (mL/h/kg)
Epoietin Alpha	6,8±0,6	19,4±2,5	8,1±0,2
Epoietin Beta	8,8±2,5	24,2±2,6	7,9±0,3
Darbepoietin	25,3±2,2	48,8±5,2	1,6±0,3
C.E.R.A	134,0±19,0	139,0±20,0	0,49±0,06

IV= intravenous; SC= subcotaneous; CL= CLearance.
C.E.R.A.= continuous erythropoietin receptor activator.

Secondary Hyperparathyroidism and Heart Valvular Disease

1. Introduction

Secondary hyperparathyroidism (sHPT) affects less than half of approximately 320.000 patients in the US who suffer from stage-V chronic kidney disease (CKD) receiving haemodialysis (HD) therapy [156]. It is characterized by elevated serum concentrations of intact parathyroid hormone (PTH), and abnormalities of serum calcium, phosphorous, and vitamin D concentrations. Insufficient treatment of sHPT has been associated with skeletal abnormalities such as renal osteodystrophy, cardiovascular complications such as myocardial hypertrophy, infections and immunoregulatory dysfunction, foot and extremity complications, and anaemia [157-160]. Patients with sHPT on HD are at increased risk for fracture, including hip fracture and mainly vascular calcification.

sHPT is an important risk factor for the development of calcifications and cardiovascular alterations in patients with CKD. In fact, the predisposition to vascular calcification was mentioned for the first time in the 19th century, since then, this topic has been the subject of many studies. This has great relevance from both the epidemiological and the clinical perspective resulting in significant morbidity, including hospitalization and mortality. Low vitamin D levels have been associated with an increased risk of vascular calcification in patients with a moderate or high risk of coronary heart disease, even with normal renal function. The prevalence of vascular calcifications in CKD patients older than 65 years of age and CV mortality is nearly 50%[160]. These percentages are only slightly lower than those observed in people undergoing HD therapy. However, the great difference is that in patients with CKD, the process of vascular calcification occurs 10–20 years earlier than in the general population and it has greater repercussions in terms of mortality. A variety of risk factors are associated with vascular calcification in dialysis patients (time on dialysis, uremic toxins, history of diabetes, inflammation), but abnormal ties in bone mineral metabolism may play a critical role. In fact, elevated serum phosphate, calcium-phosphate product, and PTH levels contribute to vascular calcification, although their roles are incompletely understood.[161].

Hyperphosphataemia may influence vascular calcification and the CV mortality risk both directly, by facilitating endothelial and intra-wall vascular calcification, and through a progressive increase in calcium deposition in the coronary arteries and heart valves, and indirectly, by worsening sHPT. Between 40 and 60% of patients undergoing dialysis have high levels of serum phosphate [162, 163].

Age, race, diabetic history, and 1,25-D levels have been related to arterial mass of coronary calcium and inversely correlated with calcium phosphate mass. In addition, a cross-sectional examination from NHANES (2001–2004) data demonstrated a inverse correlation between serum 25D levels and the prevalence of peripheral arterial disease independently of gender, age, race, and others multivariable adjustment [8]. Numerous evidences have associated arterial calcification with the presence of coronary artery disease, peripheral vascular disease, left ventricular hypertrophy and mortality in patients with CKD [158]. Furthermore, increased pulse pressure, left ventricular hypertrophy, and arrhythmias, resulting from arterial stiffness, have been proposed as potential effects of arterial calcification that may lead to CV disease and death in CKD patients.

High serum phosphate levels impair calcitriol synthesis, increase the skeletal resistance to parathyroid hormone (PTH) and also reduce PTH synthesis. These well-known consequences of hyperphosphataemia are effects on the parathyroid gland, which in turn affect bone metabolism. In addition, it is also have been that hyperphosphataemia increases parathyroid cell proliferation and may reduce expression of the calcium-sensing receptor (CaSR) [163]. These combined effects of high serum phosphate levels make serum PTH levels the most relevant indicator of sHPT severity in patients on HD.

The close relationship between elevated serum phosphate and PTH levels lead to speculate that relation between PTH levels and mortality may reproduce the effects of hyperphosphatemia.

2. Calcifications' Risk Factors in CKD Patients

CKD patients have multiple risk factors for the development of all types of calcification (Figure 7). Some of this factors can be modifiable, in the attempt of preventing extraskeletal calcification.

Arterial calcification is not a passive event as was previously believed. In fact, new evidence suggests that this process is actively regulated with both stimulatory and inhibitory factors that shares many similarities with normal bone mineralization [163].

An arbitrary division to explain the pathogenesis of vascular calcification in CKD patients has been proposed: mineral metabolism related, mineral metabolism unrelated and genetic susceptibility.

2.1. Mineral Metabolism Related

2.1.1. Increased Calcium and Phosphate Levels

Hyperphosphataemia as a consequence of decreased phosphate excretion is usually observed in advanced CKD and it is the most important modifiable risk factor for vascular calcification. Increased calcium together with calcium-phosphate product are able to strengthen the calcifying effect of hyperphosphataemia in these patients.

Increased dietary calcium intake may directly increase vascular calcification in CKD patients, and a number of studies have been shown that reversal of hyperphosphatemia and hypercalcemia using non calcium phosphate binders can induce a reduction in vascular calcification [176].

Two different mechanisms are hypothesized to explain the occurrence of vascular calcification in CKD patients with calcium-phosphate disorders [183]: a) a passive and direct calcium-phosphate precipitation in the vasculature, and b) an active induction of the expression of bone-associated genes in VSMCs [164]. In fact, it has been proposed that Increase in either calcium level, phosphorus level, or both may directly induce mineralization in human vascular smooth muscle cells in vitro via enhancing the sodium dependent phosphate cotransporter-dependent mineralization pathway. sodium-dependent phosphate cotransporter can be upregulated by both long-term elevated calcium level and hyperphophatemia. All these data indicate the importance of hyperphosphatemia and calcium load in the development of vascular calcification in CKD patients.

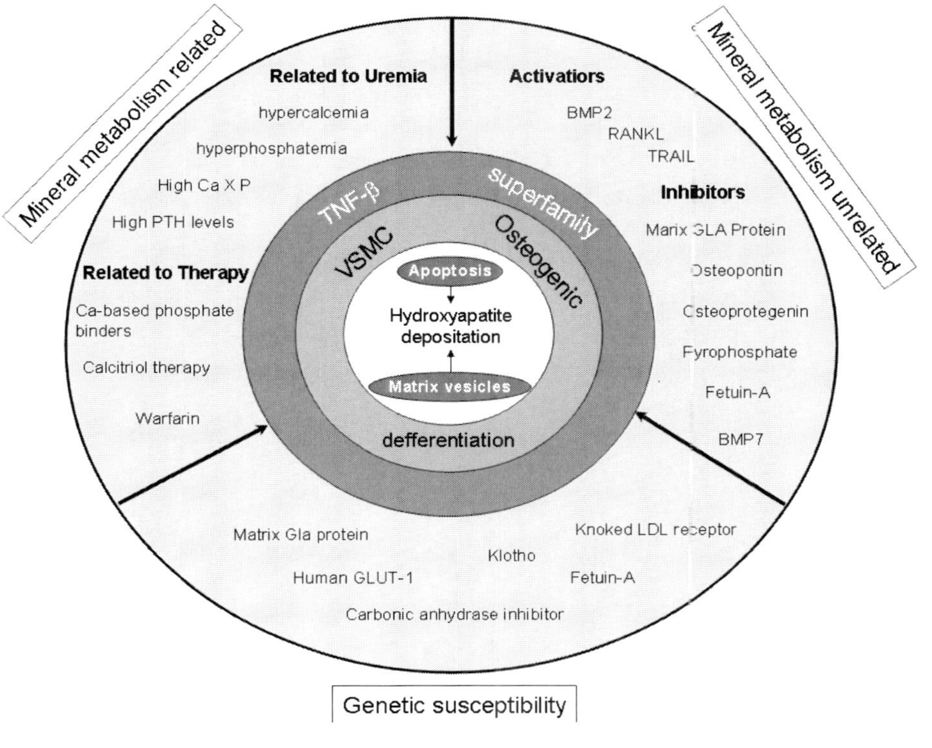

Figure 7. Mechanisms of vascular calcification in chronic kidney disease.

2.1.2. Parathyroid Hormone Level

The role of parathyroid hormone (PTH) in vascular calcification is not completely elucidated. It is possible to observe extensive vascular calcifications both in CKD patients with lower PTH levels and treated with calcium phosphate binders and in those with higher PTH levels treated with non calcium phosphate binders. In addition, any correlation has been observed between circulating PTH levels, vascular calcification score, defined according to radiographic findings of the pelvis and hands, and carotid intima-media thickness. Other authors, however, have been shown a strong correlation between coronary calcium scores and time-averaged mean serum PTH, C-reactive protein (CRP) level, Chlamydia pneumoniae seropositivity, and plasma homocysteine level [178].

Although sHPT seems to be a determinant of severity and rate of progression of vascular calcification in long-term hemodialysis patients as mentioned by certain authors, neither carotid intima-media thickness nor the number of atherosclerotic plaques were predicted by PTH level in multivariate analysis from other studies [184].

Generally, PTH and PTH-related protein are assumed to induce bone demineralization on the one hand and inhibit vascular calcification on the other hand, in concert with other inhibitors of mineralization of VSMCs such as fetuin-A, matrix Gla protein, and vitamin K [185,186]. To summarize, most authorities suggest that PTH may have a protective effect against vascular calcification, and the severity of vascular calcification may increase in conditions of adynamic bone disease and low PTH.

2.1.3. Vitamin D

The impact of vitamin D on vascular calcification is not clearly known. Vitamin D receptors are contained in several human tissues and active vitamin D metabolites can be synthesized locally both in endothelial cells and VSMC which contains 1α-hydroxylase [188,189]. A negative correlation between 1,25-dihydroxy vitamin D3 level and coronary calcification have been shown in CKD patients with high risk for coronary artery disease[190]. In addition, it is well known a increased vascular calcification as the result of active vitamin D therapy in uremic patients.

Inflammatory cytokines may play an important role in vascular calcification. Tumor necrosis factor (TNF-α) may induce 1α-hydroxylase suggesting a novel autocrine/paracrine role for the enzyme, possibly as a modulator of endothelial cell adhesion. In patients with advanced CKD, carotid intima-media thickness and calcification scores shown a U-shaped distribution across 1,25-dihydroxyvitamin D levels, thus patients with both low and high 1,25-dihydroxyvitamin D had significantly greater carotid intima-media thickness and calcification scores than those with normal levels. On the other hands, low 1,25-dihydroxyvitamin D levels were also associated with higher levels of high-sensitivity CRP, strengthening the hypothesis of a link between vascular calcification and inflammation.

Vitamin D plus vitamin K supplementation may improve elastic properties of the common carotid artery probably through increased activity of matrix Gla protein, which is a potent inhibitor of vascular calcification and dependent on vitamin D and Vitamin for its action.

In hemodialysis patients direct correlation have been found between extension of vascular calcification and circulating vitamin D concentration. In addition, there are a good relationship between cumulative calcitriol intake and active vitamin D metabolite levels and left ventricular mass index [191].

In a animal model of secondary hyperparathyroidism, both calcitriol and cinacalcet have been successful in control of hyperparathyroidism. However, only calcitriol-induced hypercalcemia increased calcium - phosphorus product and vascular calcification. Furthermore, high-dose calcitriol treatment in uremic rats with sHPT could induce hypertension, LVH, and diffuse aortic intimal and medial calcification in the absence of hypercalcemia and increased calcium-phosphorus product, compared to vehicle-treated uremic rats and sham operated rats. Others studies have also shown that fibroblast growth factor 23 and Klotho knockout mice develop widespread soft tissue and vascular calcification due to uninhibited production of active vitamin D, hypercalcemia and hyperphosphatemia [192, 193].

Overall, this data seems that there is a delicate balance between the protective effect of vitamin D on cardiovascular system and its vascular calcifying effect. This phenomena may itself occur with either high or low doses of vitamin D supplementation.

2.2. Mineral Metabolism Unrelated

Molecular mechanisms: Various proteins involved in osteogenesis have been shown to be present in VSMCs and atherosclerotic lesions such as osteopontin, BMP2 and matrix Gla protein. Vascular calcification is a complex process resulting in a combination between stimulating proteins such as BMP2 and receptor activator of nuclear factor-kappa B (RANK) ligand and inhibitory proteins such as matrix Gla protein, BMP7, osteoprotegerin, fetuin-A, and osteopontin [199, 200].

Vascular calcification starts with formation of matrix vesicles, which are small extracellular membrane-derived particles selectively located in the matrix of the bone, cartilage, and predentin. These particles contain calcium-binding proteins and phosphatases for nucleation of hydroxyapatite. The vesicles are the initial site of calcification in all skeletal tissue, and hydroxyapatite crystals are generated in them during a phosphatase-dependent phase 1 mineralization. Phase 2 of mineralization begins with breakdown of matrix vesicle membranes, exposing preformed hydroxyapatite to the extracellular fluid, after which mineral crystal proliferation is regulated by extracellular conditions [195, 196].

Another important factor in initiation of vascular calcification is apoptosis of VSMCs [199]. In fact, the role of apoptosis in pathogenesis of human atherosclerotic lesions was further confirmed by a number of studies. Apoptosis can be induced by the interaction of VSMCs with inflammatory cells that express cell surface death ligands or secrete proapoptotic cytokines such as TNF-α. Apoptosis precedes vascular calcification in vitro, and VSMC-derived apoptotic bodies can concentrate and crystallize calcium. It has been observed that vascular calcification was initiated by the release of membrane-bound matrix vesicles from living VSMCs and also by the release of apoptotic bodies from dying cells. This situation could not happen in the presence of serum with mineralization inhibitors, such as fetuin-A and matrix Gla protein [197]. On the other hand, vesicles released by VSMCs after prolonged exposure to calcium and phosphorus contained preformed basic calcium phosphate and calcified extensively.

Plasma Proteins. There are a number of proteins involved in vascular calcification acting either as inhibitors or inducers of this process. Matrix Gla protein, which is a bone matrix protein with 5 to 6 residues of the vitamin K-dependent amino acid, gamma-carboxyglutamic acid, is mainly known as an inhibitor of calcification by inhibiting mesenchymal cell differentiation to the osteogenic lineage by preventing the action of the potent osteogenic and chondrogenic differentiation factor, BMP2 [203].

In osteoporotic mice lacking matrix Gla protein have been observed spontaneous arteries and cartilages calcification. Thus, matrix Gla protein may be required to both promote normal bone formation and inhibit vascular calcification. Matrix Gla protein gamma-carboxylation is a vitamin K-dependent process. Therefore, vitamin K deficiency can inhibit matrix Gla protein action and enhance vascular calcification. However, no correlation have been found between matrix Gla protein and coronary artery or aortic calcification score in dialysis patients [197].

In dialysis patients low levels of vitamin K have been shown, and consequently decreased level of circulating matrix Gla protein has been proposed as a predictor of mortality. However, outcomes improvements have not been observed after vitamin K supplementation.

Another important matrix protein with inhibitory capacity of calcification is Osteopontin [203], which is an acidic phosphoprotein normally found in mineralized tissues such as bones and teeth, as well as in the kidney and epithelial linings of the body. Osteopontin acts through self-aggregation and adhesion to apatite crystals through specific amino acid moieties. Osteopontin is able to inhibit calcification in bovine aortic smooth muscle culture media. In dialysis patients Osteopontin levels are associated with the presence and severity of coronary artery calcification.

Fetuin-A [200-202] is also an important calcification inhibitor. This protein interacts directly with matrix vesicle release and may thus modulate vascular calcification processes locally and at early stages. The "calciprotein particles," which is constituted by Fetuin-A molecules form stable colloidal spheres with calcium and phosphorus, inhibit hydroxyapatite precipitation, decreases macrophage activation and also release of proinflammatory cytokines, antagonizes the action of transforming growth factor-β, and opsonises apoptotic bodies and promotes their phagocytosis.

In dialysis patients Fetuin-A levels are significantly lower and this has been correlated with higher rates of vascular calcification, cardiovascular mortality, malnutrition and inflammation states. Fetuin-A has been proposed as both a calcification inhibitor protein and a negative acute-phase reactant, as a link between inflammation atherosclerosis in patients with CKD.

Osteoprotegerin which is a glycoprotein and member of TNF receptor family, inhibits osteoclast maturation and protects bone from normal osteoclast remodeling. It functions as a soluble decoy receptor for RANK ligand (osteoprotegerin ligand) and shares homologies with other members of the TNF receptor superfamily [203]. The role of Osteoprotegerin in the genesis of vascular calcification is complex and is under investigation.

There are other proteins that working in this context such as BMP2 and BMP7 which role in decrease vascular calcification is under investigation.

2.3. Genetic Susceptibility

In animal models several genetic studies have shown susceptibility of vascular calcification. Myocardial cell necrosis and calcification have been demonstrated in inbred mice with a single major locus Dyscalc, located on proximal chromosome 7 in a region syntenic with human chromosomes 19q13 and 11p15. In apolipoprotein E deficient mice, osteopontin deficiency may attenuate atherosclerosis and aggravate vascular calcification. In low density lipoprotein (LDL)-receptor deficient mice, atherosclerosis may prevent by inhibitory factor deficiency of macrophage migration, and spontaneous calcification of arteries and cartilage in mice lacking matrix Gla protein, In addition in vitro enhanced susceptibility of smooth muscle cells deficient in osteopontin to calcification. Further examples of susceptibility of vascular calcification are given for mice knocked out in the membrane protein Klotho, carbonic anhydrase inhibitor, or Fetuin A (an important calcification inhibitor protein)[169,170, 172].

In human studies, increased vascular calcification has been associated with increased platelet reactivity due to single nucleotide polymorphism on chromosome 9p21.3 [172].

In diabetic patients a subclinical atherosclerosis has been associated with lipoxygenase gene pathway variations and parathyroid gene AA variant is more prevalent among patients with degenerative aortic stenosis calcification. Interestingly a single nucleotide polymorphism of bone morphogenetic protein (BMP) have been associated with inverse relationships between bone mineralization and calcification in the coronary, carotid, and abdominal aorta in a diabetes patients [173].

Despite many other genetic predispositions to vascular calcification have also been described in normal kidney function population, there are few evidences available in patients with CKD. In non - diabetic patients with CKD and vascular calcification, there is a higher prevalence of polymorphism in a glucose transporter gene (GLUT-1 XbaI). High intracellular glucose concentration has been found in clones human cells with over-expression the GLUT-1 transporter. It has bee hypothesized that high intracellular glucose together with uremic factors may play a role in vascular calcification by transforming VSMCs into osteoblast-like cells.

3. Secondary Hyperparathyroidism and Cardiovascular Damage

It is universally recognized that CKD patients have a dramatically higher incidence of cardiovascular morbidity and mortality compared to the general population. In fact, CVD mortality is 10 to 70 times greater in the dialysis patients than in the general population. In the last decade, several studies pointed out that vascular calcification is a major cause of cardiovascular disease in the dialysis population [204].

In dialysis patients, aortic stiffness, represented by aortic pulse wave velocity and carotid distensibility, are strong independent predictors of cardiovascular and all-cause mortality. In fact, carotid pulse pressure, as a measure of central pulse pressure, and mostly the disappearance of pulse pressure amplification have been demonstrated as strong independent predictors of all-cause, including cardiovascular, mortality. In addition, lack of aortic pulse wave velocity decrease consequently to drug-induced reduction in blood pressure have been found a significant predictor of cardiovascular death in CKD patients [205].

Hemodialysis patients with arterial intimal and medial calcification had a significantly shorter survival compared to patients with intimal calcification rather than those patients without calcifications [207]. Thus, arterial medial calcification seems to be a strong prognostic marker of all-cause and cardiovascular mortality in dialysis patients, independently of classical atherogenic factors. Furthermore, the presence of extent of vascular calcifications, detected by ultrasonography and abdominopelvic radiography seems to be an other strong predictors of cardiovascular and all-cause mortality [208].

Even after kidney transplantation, vascular calcification is an important determinant of cardiovascular events. In fact, aortic calcification, detecting by electron beam computed tomography, has been proposed as predict future cardiovascular events in kidney transplant recipients [208].

In the last decade several study and clinical trials have shown high prevalence of the LVH in the patients with CKD. Further extension of this link is given by the finding of more than 80% prevalence of concentric and eccentric LVH among patients with CKD not yet in dialysis therapy [209]. Most of patients, nearly to 80%, of initiating dialysis presented with LVH determined with echocardiography.

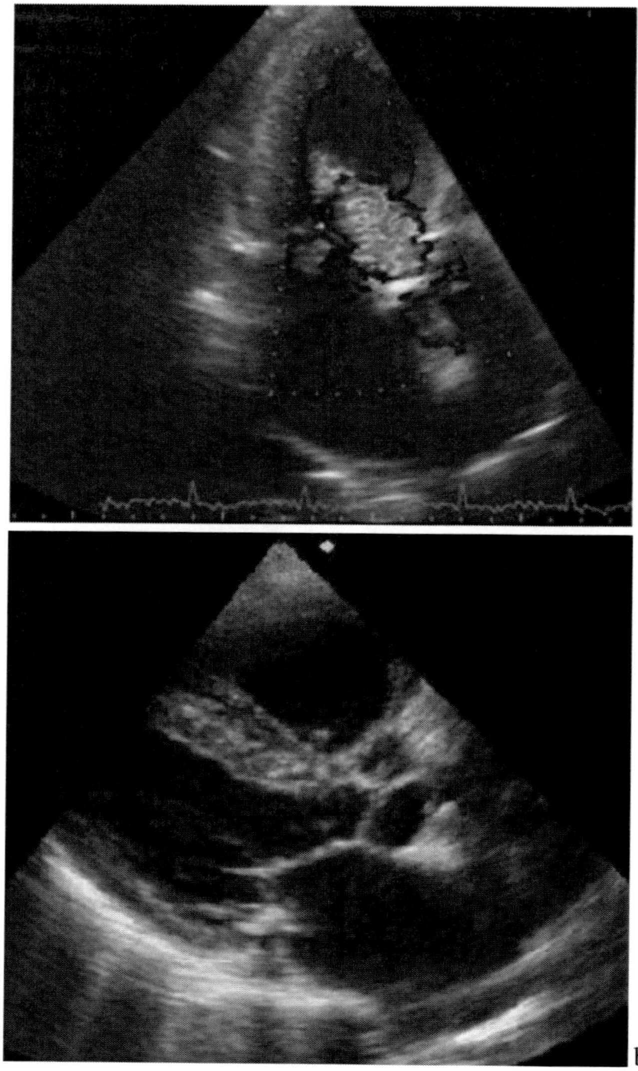

a)

b)

a) Aortic valve calcification with moderate-severe stenosis component.
b) Mitral valve calcification involving the prevalently the posterior leaflets.

Figure 8. A: Echocardiogram shows typical Aortic valve calcification with moderate-severe stenosis component and B: Mitral valve calcification involving the prevalently the posterior leaflets in two hemodialysis patients diagnosed by cardiac ultrasonographic measurement.

The relationship between high levels of PTH and LVH has been observed that surgical correction of advances sHPT with parathyroidectomy in CKD patients induced to a significant improvement of left ventricular ejection fraction and function [207].

Hyperphosphatemia and hypercalcemia have been shown to promote calcification of the vasculature, myocardium, and cardiac valves. Vascular calcification manifested in reduced vessel wall elasticity, increased intima-media layer thickness, and enhanced pulse-wave velocity—has been linked to LVH—and occurs with increased severity in dialysis patients versus non-CKD patients.

Aortic valve calcification (AVC) or mitral annulus calcification (MAC) has been considered to be a chronic, non - inflammatory degenerative process that occurs predominantly in elderly patients. Recent studies reported a high prevalence of valvular and vascular calcification in patients with CKD. Other than aging, deregulation of mineral metabolism with a high calcium load and the resulting poor calcium-phosphorus balance are suggested to be largely responsible for the excessive valvular and vascular calcification in this population. The recent demonstration of a significant association between C-reactive protein and valvular calcification suggests that calcification in patients with CKD may not simply be a passive degenerative process but rather may involve active inflammation.

In large non-CKD population cohort studies, AVC and MAC have been associated with increased cardiovascular mortality and morbidity specially in diabetic patients. Furthermore, higher serum phosphate levels within the normal range were associated with valvular and annular calcification in a community-based cohort of older adults. Thus, circulating phosphate levels may play a novel risk factor for calcific aortic valve disease.

In a recent study, MAC has been associated with increased mortality and significant coronary artery disease in a group of renal transplant candidates. These patients have increased LV cavity size, poorer LV systolic function, higher LV filling pressures compared to patients without MAC.

In patients with CKD treated with conservative rather than with dialysis therapy, more attention needs to be given to the control of sHPT reduce the risk of cardiovascular morbidity and mortality in dialysis patients.

3.1. Diagnosis of Cardiovascular Calcification

The gold standard for diagnosis of vascular calcification would be histological examination of the arterial samples, which is not clinically feasible. Other recommended diagnostic techniques is electron beam computed tomography, which is more of research interest and not accessible in most centers of the world. Cardiac ultrasonographic measurement (Figure 8), pulse wave velocity, carotid intima-media thickness and plain radiography of the abdominal aorta would be more feasible to perform and economically more sustainable in most dialysis. The Kidney Disease Improving Global Outcomes [209] guidelines suggest a lateral abdominal radiography or an echocardiography for detection of the presence or absence of vascular or valvular calcification, in stages 3 to 5 CKD patients. However, specific screening for presence and severity of vascular calcification is not yet recommended by many authorities due to uncertainty on the sensitivity and specificity of the recommended screening methods, cost versus benefit of these methods, and lack of effective treatment modalities.

3.2. Treatment Strategies to Prevent Cardiovascular Calcification

A positive interaction has been found between dosage of calcium-based phosphate binders and bone activity. In fact, calcium load has been shown to significantly influence on aortic calcifications and stiffening in the presence of adynamic bone disease.

Development of coronary artery calcification has been associated with lower trabecular bone volume and, on the other hand, improvement in bone turnover has been correlated with lower rate of progression of coronary artery calcification.

Therefore, many studies now denote the strategy of employing non-calcium-based phosphate binders to prevent and / or regress vascular calcification.

In fact, an increase in median absolute calcium score in coronary arteries and aorta, measured by electron beam tomography has been found in calcium-based phosphate binders compared with those treated with non-calcium-based phosphate binders CKD patients. Similarly, decreased levels of total and LDL cholesterol, apolipoprotein B, β2-microglobulin, and highly sensitivity CRP, and increased level of high-density lipoprotein have been observed in patient treated with sevelamer but not in those treated with calcium-based binders dialysis patients [210]. Even if these data have been also confirmed in other trials, there is not an unanimous position about this issue. In a large study including more than 1000 hemodialysis patients followed for up to 45 months, the overall mortality was not significantly reduced by sevelamer compared with calcium-based phosphate binders, except for patients older than 65 years of age, in whom sevelamer reduced the risk of death. Also, a recent systematic review on clinical efficacy and safety of sevelamer in dialysis patients could not show any evidence that sevelamer reduced all-cause mortality, cardiovascular mortality, the frequency of symptomatic bone disease, or health - related quality of life.

Cinacalcet [212] has also been tested in terms of its impact and prevention on vascular calcification. In a combined analysis of 4 similar studies including 1184 advanced CKD patients with hyperphosphatemia and secondary hyperparathyroidism (697 patients on cinacalcet and 487 on placebo), Cinacalcet significantly reduced cardiovascular hospitalization compared with placebo. Data of the ADVANCE clinical trial [211], clearly shows that therapy with cinacalcet plus low-dose vitamin D sterols may attenuate vascular and cardiac valve calcification in CKD patients on hemodialysis therapy with moderate to severe sHPT. The results of the EVOLVE trial may further delineate this issue, by examining the effect of cinacalcet on all-cause and cardiovascular mortality and morbidity, peripheral vascular disease, and stroke in hyperparathyroid maintenance hemodialysis patients.

Other medications suggested for attenuation of vascular calcification in CKD patients are bisphophonates, BMP7 that has been investigated in murine models of vascular calcification, anti-RANK ligand therapy, and teriparatide used for inhibition of vascular calcification in diabetic LDL-deficient mice.

Atherosclerosis, Chronic Inflammation and CKD

Since the late 1990s elevated circulating levels of C-reactive protein has been reported in patients with end-stage renal disease, an atherogenic, wasted phenotype and with poor outcome [213, 214].

Chronic inflammation clearly plays a key role in both the initiation and progression of many chronic diseases, including chronic renal failure, diabetes mellitus and cardiovascular disease. Although the various chronic inflammatory processes may appear to be diverse, they involve similar cellular activities and utilize similar signaling pathways. Firstly inflammation in chronic diseases appears to be chronic yet from the onset, starting with infiltration of tissues by monocytes and macrophages, [215] which is in contrast to the initial accumulation of polymorphonuclear leukocytes seen in acute inflammation.

It is therefore likely that the factors that initiate and regulate chronic inflammatory processes differ from those involved in acute inflammation. In fact even the development of atherosclerosis was associated to infection by various microbial pathogens [216-218], in many chronic diseases no pathogens have been identified, with the evidence that these processes proceed in sterile settings. In atherosclerosis, shear stress can modulate gene expression of endothelial cells, increasing permeability to low-density lipoprotein (LDL) and promoting monocyte infiltration [217-218]. Modified LDLs can promote the formation of foam cells, which together with other mediators activate innate immunity. The innate immune system represents the earliest barrier to invading pathogens and provides important cues for the adaptive immunity that follows. It recognizes the repetitive molecular structures of pathogens, which are known as pathogen-associated molecular patterns (PAMPs), through pattern recognition receptors (PRRs) [219].

Cells of the innate immune system, such as macrophages, express a variety of PRRs, including the Toll-like receptors (TLRs). Upon recognition of a PAMP, TLRs activate several signaling molecules, among which the nuclear factor κ B (NF-κB) pathway is the most distinctive. The resultant signaling causes innate immune cells to be activated to destroy the pathogen and/or pathogen infected cells, and may also lead to activation of adaptive immunity.

Damage to tissues and cells can also be caused by trauma induced by physical or chemical insults. The resultant damaged or dying cells release endogenous molecules called damage/ danger-associated molecular patterns (DAMPs), which activate the immune system in a fashion analogous to PAMPs [220]. It has also been proposed that modified endogenous molecules, such as oxidized lipoproteins, serve as DAMPs [221,222] In addition, it was recently shown that cholesterol crystals induce inflammation by stimulating the NLRP3 inflammasome [223].

In this way, modified self molecules, the production of which does not necessarily require cell death, may serve as danger signals that activate PRRs and innate immune responses. Within adipose tissue, proinflammatory cytokines produced by macrophages can activate lipolysis and increase release of FFAs from adipocytes. These saturated FFAs, in turn, can activate macrophages and then it has therefore been proposed that adipocytes and macrophages form a vicious link that enhances inflammation in obese adipose tissue [224].

These findings are exceptionally remarkable because they suggest that nutrient molecules can directly activate the innate immune response, under sterile conditions. Finally, although innate immune responses are central to chronic inflammatory processes, the adaptive and innate immune systems appear to intrinsically interact to control inflammatory processes [225].

It is easy to imagine acute inflammation as initiated and employed as an adaptive and protective mechanism against insults. On the other side even chronic inflammatory processes may also have essential homeostatic and protective functions. In fact, when DAMPs are generated by tissue damage and cell death, chronic inflammation and clearance of dead cells by macrophages is essential to prevent further release of intracellular materials and to restrain inflammation. In line with these hypothesis, mice showing inadequate engulfment of apoptotic cells develop a systemic lupus erythematosus-like autoimmune disease [226].

In addition to TLRs, natural antibodies secreted by B-1 innate-type B cells help to maintain tissue homeostasis, recognizing oxidized lipids and antigens expressed by apoptotic cells [227], facilitating uptake of apoptotic cells by macrophages [228] and exerting atheroprotective effects [229].

Within adipose tissue, inflammation can be activated under physiological conditions by both feeding and fasting. Fasting activates lipolysis and increases the release of FFAs from adipocytes, which recruit macrophages to the adipose tissue [232], and then these cells phagocytise the excess lipids. Importantly, these processes can be activated by a 24-h fast, as well as by weight loss induced by 30% caloric restriction, suggesting the macrophage accumulation is an embedded physiological program for the maintenance of homeostasis. Taken together, these findings suggest that in many cases of chronic disease, chronic inflammatory processes are initially activated to protect cells and tissue from stress. Clarifying how these processes, which are initially beneficial, become pathological will be important for understanding the mechanisms underlying chronic inflammatory diseases.

The possibility of treating this condition has been much discussed. Several small studies have implied that various nutritional and pharmacological treatment strategies have beneficial effects on surrogate markers of inflammation. On the other hand, although inflammatory markers persistently predict outcome in dialysis patients or following kidney transplantation, few studies have studied the effect of these interventions on outcome [214].

Small studies reported encouraging results on the levels of inflammatory biomarkers following intervention with gamma-tocopherol [230], soy [231], green tea [232], cholecalciferol [233] and sevelamer [234]. When a RCT tested on 2776 hemodialysis patients the effects of rosuvastatin versus placebo [235], no effect on mortality was observed despite a small reduction of CRP following statin treatment. However, as the interaction between CRP and the effect of rosuvastatin was not checked, we do not know if the effects of statins on the outcome differ between inflamed and uninflamed dialysis patients. Small studies tested the hypothesis that anti-cytokine therapy could affect surrogate biomarkers of inflammation, morbidity, and mortality in chronic pathologies.

Salsalate (a prodrug of salicylic acid with inhibitory effects on the NF-κB pathway), Anakinra (an IL-1 receptor antagonist) and an IL-1β-specific antibody were tested in T2D patients [236-238]. The positive results of these studies are consistent with the concept of targeting inflammation to treat T2D.

Large clinical trials of the TNF-α antagonist, etanercept, in patients with NYHA classes II–IV heart failure failed to show a beneficial effect on the incidences of death and hospitalization. Similarly, the monoclonal antibody, infliximab, failed to show a therapeutic benefit. There are several possibilities as to why these clinical trials failed: [213] the dose and timing of treatment were not sufficient to inhibit TNF-α; [214] the biological agents had unknown detrimental side effects and/or intrinsic toxicity; and [215] treatment interfered with other drug treatments [239]. Although these explanations are all plausible, it is also known that TNF-α contributes to cardioprotection related to ischemic conditioning.

This means that the choice of timing, dose and subjects very likely affected the therapeutic consequences. Clearly, a more detailed understanding of the mechanisms underlying chronic inflammation is needed, particularly in relation to the temporal progression of disease processes. It will also be important to determine how inflammatory processes become activated in multiple tissues if we are to understand the accumulation of tissue dysfunctions often seen in patients with chronic disease.

A recent small pilot study (only 10 subjects) did not observe significant effects on inflammatory biomarkers on dialysis patients randomly assigned to receive either the tumour necrosis factor-alpha (TNF-a) antagonist etanercept or placebo twice weekly for 44 weeks [240]. Thus, larger studies are now needed to test the effects of selective anti-TNF, IL-1, and IL-6 therapies, respectively, not only on inflammatory and nutritional surrogate markers but also on morbidity and outcome. No doubt, the major problem in such a RCT will be to select the patients with persistent non-infectious uremic inflammation.

Until adequately powered RCTs have been performed with anti-inflammatory treatment strategies, no specific pharmacological treatment recommendations for uremic inflammation can be advocated. However, clinicians should be aware of the strong association between persistent inflammation and outcome before carefully evaluating and treating the possible causes, unrelated (infectious and inflammatory complications, peridontitis, and ischemic heart disease) or related to dialysis (materials biocompatibility, residual renal function, vascular access infections, impure dialysate, volume overload).

Cardio-Renal Syndromes

1. Introduction

Cardio-Renal Syndrome (CRS) is actually used to define several clinical conditions of heart and kidney failure [241]. Functional dialogue between heart and kidney, in normal condition and during disease, is complex and fascinating. This virtuous duo plays a marvellous melody, with the heart delivering fluids to all body districts, while kidney surveys composition and volume of these fluids.

The definition of cardio-renal syndrome has been often used to describe only chronic renal failure due to chronic heart failure. Actually this misunderstanding involves in a partial vision of the problem preventing complete analysis of all clinical situations in which cardiac and renal dysfunction overlap.

An effective classification has been proposed in 2008 by Consensus Group of Acute Dialysis Quality Group [241], as reported in table 7.

According to this classification, CRS is mainly divided in two fundamental groups: cardio-renal and reno-cardiac syndromes, on the basis of *primum movens* of disease. Further subdivision in each group, defined as acute or chronic, is according to the modality of onset of disease.

Fifth group collects all CRS due to systemic diseases, breaking the elegant design of this classification, in our opinion.

It's important to underline that cardiac disease related to chronic renal failure (CRS type IV) is only one of the 5 types of CRS and that there are at least other three forms that are completely different from this one. These CRS types are due to primary cardiac diseases (acute or chronic, CRS type I and II) or acute renal disease (CRS type III).

Table 7. CRS Classification

Type	Denomination	Description	Example
1	Acute cardiorenal	Heart failure leading to AKD	Acute coronary syndrome leading to acute heart and kidney failure
2	Chronic cardiorenal	Chronic heart failure leading to kidney failure	Chronic heart failure
3	Acute nephrocardiac	AKD leading to acute heart failure	Uremic cardiomiopathy AKD - related
4	Chronic nephrocardiac	Chronic kidney disease leading to heart failure	Left ventricular hyperthrophy and diastolic heart failure due to kidney failure
5	Secondary	Systemic disease leading to heart and kidney failure	Sepsis, vasculitis, diabetes mellitus

Some criticism have been raised to this classification, regarding the right to use the term "syndrome" before the simultaneous presence of multiple diseases without any multiplicative effect in terms of risk. It is our opinion that this criticisms do not affect the clinical utility of this classification, revolutionary in the capacity to clear to physicians that cardiorenal syndrome is not only uremic cardiomiopathy.

2. Diagnosis

2.1. CRS Type I

A typical form of *CRS type I* (acute cardiac disease inducing acute renal failure) is related to acute coronary syndrome. Incidence of acute renal failure in patients hospitalized for acute myocardial infarction is about 2-4% [242]. It is then important to promptly recognize this form of CRS and correct cardiologic and nephrological aspects of syndrome. This kind of patient is in an intensive cardiological setting, and he is at risk for developing acute coronary syndrome, sepsis, acute valvular pathology or pericarditis.

CRS type I has not typical and exclusive ECG patterns, even if crucial informations can be obtained from the ECG trace.

Patients typically show fluids overload, characterized by high voltages in QRS complex and prominent T waves, while even ST – T tract asymmetric elevation or diphasic T – waves are described less frequently.

INegative T – waves in precordial derivations can subtend to coronary syndromes or pericardial effusions. In the second case it is frequent to register low voltages in peripheral derivations.

Typically this patient will not present ultrasonographic and clinical stigmata of chronic renal failure.

Ultrasonography could early detect and allow follow-up for presence of:

1. any myocardial kinetic abnormality, indicating an ischemic condition particularly if rapidly worsening and left ventricular hypertrophy (Figure 1).

2. valvular stenosis and insufficiency, particularly if rapidly worsening (like in case of endocarditis);
3. pericardial effusions;
4. normal inspiratory collapse of inferior vena cava;
5. aortic aneurisms or dissection.

CRS diagnosis is a field in which application of ultrasound imaging techniques is particularly helpful [255].

For the clinician, there are three fundamental advantages in the direct management of ultrasound imaging: no needs of invasive techniques, good cost/effectiveness ratio and wide staircase available technology.

Echocardiography represents one of most spreading techniques in cardiological practice, as we can consider it such a complement to patient's bedside examination.

On the other hand, renal ultrasound provides many informations about kidney structure with special focus on size and echogenicity of kidney parenchimal architecture.

2.1. CRS Type II

In *CRS type II,* chronic and cardio-renal, patient is typically affected by chronic congestive heart failure. About 3% of patients hospitalized for congestive heart failure present renal failure with 22% rate of mortality [243-246]. Clinical outcome of these patients gets worse even with small increasing of serum creatinine, independently from pre-existent chronic renal failure and from left ventricular dysfunction severity [243-246].Patients with congestive heart failure GFR has a predictive value as ejection fraction and NYHA functional class [246,247].

These patients are insidious, because they are not clearly diagnosed often belonging to low specialized Units where patients are affected by several diagnosis.

Fluids overload, characterized by high voltages in QRS complex and prominent T waves, while even unspecific ST – T tract anomalies or diphasic T – waves are described less frequently.

Hypertensive patients, in presence of ventricular hypertrophy, typically show similar QRS high complexes and unspecific repolarisation phase abnormalities.

In chronic cardio-renal syndrome, pathological Q waves, elevation of ST tract or negative T – waves in precordial derivations can subtend to ischemic cardiopathy.

In presence of pericardial effusions, T wave usually is negative and peaked, with short ST tracts. In this case it is frequent to register low voltages in peripheral derivations.

Ultrasonographic examination will keep attention to:

1. renal ultrasonographic clues of "*chronicity*".
2. high atrial volumes or areas as indices of volume overload.
3. low ejection fraction.
4. right chamber dilation, high estimated pulmonary arterial pressure (PAPs) and lower tricuspid annulus plane systolic excursion (TAPSE).
5. pericardial effusions (Figure 3 - 4).
6. chronic valvular pathology, with particular attention to valvular calcifications.

2.2. CRS Type III

CRS type III, acute and reno-cardiac is quite frequent in nephrological emergency setting. In these patients volume overload due to acute renal failure leads to acute heart failure; ECG and echocardiography imaging can be insidious and silent.

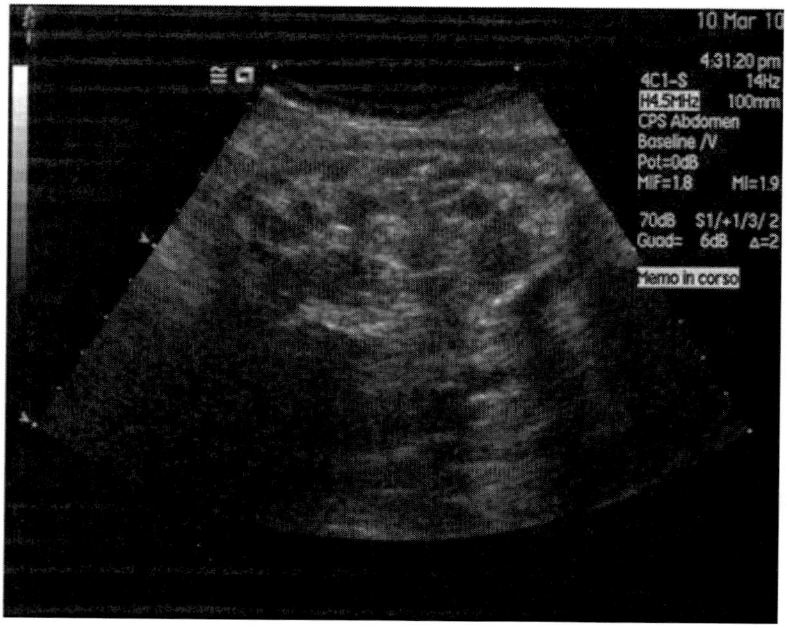

Figure 9. Kidney in end – stage renal disease (marked hyperechogenicity of kidney cortical with reduction of cortico – medullar ratio).

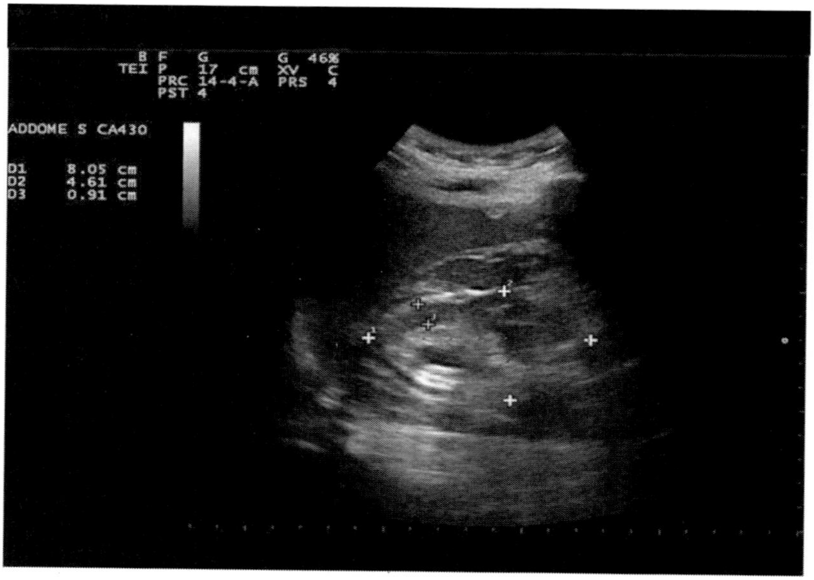

Figure 10. End – stage kidney with marked hyperechogenicity and reduction of cortico – medullar ratio.

Kidney's size and its parenchymal echogenicity provide primary features to discern between acute and chronic nephropathies always remembering that kidney volume and longitudinal diameter correlate with patient's height and body surface [256, 257] and that many CKD patients show enlarged kidneys (e.g. early stages of diabetic nephropathy, HIV-related glomerulonephritis, cast nephropathy). Hyper echoic renal cortical with medullary hypoechogenicity and low cortico – medullary ratio, is quite predictive of chronic nephropathy [256, 257] (Figure 9, Figure 10). On the other hand, cortical hyperechogenicity can be sometimes evident in acute tubular necrosis (Figure 11) or Systemic Erhytematous Lupus nephritis [256, 257]. Renal ultrasound is obviously crucial in differential diagnosis of obstructive nephropaties with particular attention to:

1. high atrial volumes or areas as indices of volume overload;
2. pleural or pericardial effusion;
3. lung comets;
4. renal parenchimal echogenicity;
5. renal volume;
6. urinary tracts dilation;
7. inversed diastolic flow at interlobar renal arteries.

2.3. CRS Type IV

CRS type IV represents most widely diagnosed CRS type by clinicians with more available epidemiological data. About 50% of causes of death in end stage renal disease are due to cardiovascular events, 10-20 times more frequent than in general population [243-246]. About 50% of patients undergoing hemodialytic treatment present an acute cardiovascular event within two years from the beginning of extracorporeal renal replacement therapy.

Uremic patient are at high risk of intra-dialytic arrhythmias, as like of sudden death.

QT, or better QTc (correcting QT for the heart rate, according to Bazett equation) prolongation or dispersion are typically used to measure and monitor this risk. A strict electrocardiographic survey of this patients is then highly useful.

In this setting, ultrasonographic monitoring verifies dry weight targets and investigates dyspnoea in uremic patients [259, 260, 261]. Ultrasonographic examination points up on:

1. high atrial volumes or areas as indices of volume overload.
2. pleural or pericardial effusion (Figure 3, 4).
3. lung comets.
4. valvular calcifications.
5. clues of right dysfunction (high PAPs, low TAPSE, right chambers dilation).

Type V CRS represents a container of different chronic pathologies causing CRS, ranging from sepsis to Type 2 Diabetes Mellitus. In every conditions listed above, physician will find comfortable analyze clinical pictures as acute or chronic, reno-cardiac or cardio-renal, and he can apply what previous described.

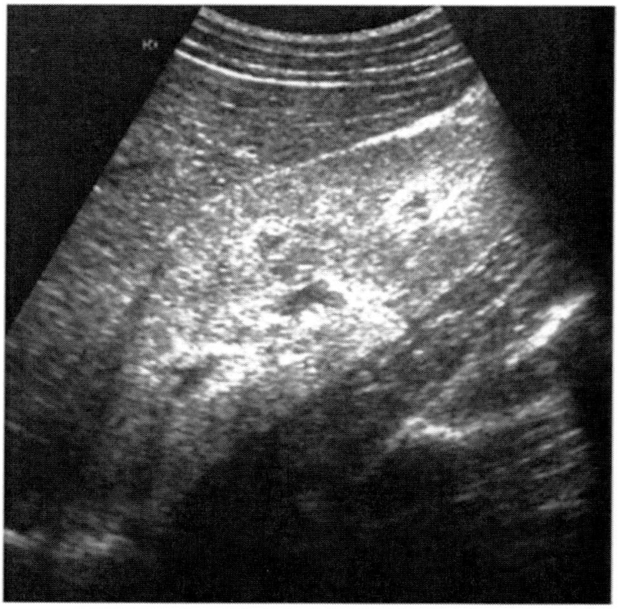

Figure 11. Kidney hyperechogenicity in Acute tubular necrosis.

3. Management

3.1. Management of Heart Congestive Symptoms

First of all we have to manage congestive symptoms such as dyspnoea and peripheral edema. Loop diuretics represent first – line pharmacological agents to control congestive symptoms [262] but they have carefully employed because of association with electrolyte abnormalities, neurohormonal activation and worsening of kidney function.

Vasodilators, such as intravenous nitroglycerin, are recommended in acute heart failure patients without hypotension or severe valvular disease [262].

Nesiritide, an analogue of human brain natriuretic peptide, was tested to determine whether was superior to placebo in reducing heart failure related hospitalization but outcomes were not positive [263].

Ultrafiltration can be helpful in removing volume overload in symptomatic heart failure patients refractory to diuretic therapy obtaining greater fluids removal and lower hospitalization rates [264].

Inotropic agents have to be considered in patients with signs and symptoms of tissues hypoperfusion and low – output clinical conditions. Dobutamine increases renal blood flow as it increases cardiac output [262]

3.2. Management of Renal Dysfunction in Chronic Heart Failure

Several drugs can be employed to manage kidney function in chronic heart failure but most of them can worse renal function. Prospective studies have tried to catch some evidence about impact of AHA/ACC guidelines recommendations in management of chronic heart failure (ACEi, ARB, Beta – blockers, aldosterone antagonists, cardiac resynchronization therapy, implantable cardioverter defibrillator, anticoagulation if atrial fibrillation/flutter) on renal function. Multivariate analysis showed that the severity of CKD was an independent predictor of adherence to ACEI/ARB; treatment with ACEI improves ventricular function (as evidenced by an increased ejection fraction and decreased ventricular size) and patient well-being, reduces hospital admission for worsening HF, and increases survival. This therapy should be used in all patients with symptomatic HF and a LVEF < 40% [22]. As it is common to observe a significant increase in the serum creatinine concentration (>0.3 mg/dL) within the initiation of treatment with ACEI, renal function should be closely monitored. Treatment with ACEI must be interrupted if creatinine serum concentration rises above 3.5 mg/dL. ARB may be considered as an alternative in patients who do not tolerate ACEI. The influence on cardiorenal protection of RAAS dual blockade, when an ARB is used in conjunction with an ACEI, has also been analyzed in several trials. Among patients with HF, combination therapy was associated with further impairment in kidney function [265]. An aldosterone antagonist should be added to treatment in symptomatic patients with HF and an LVEF < 35% [262].

The Canadian Cardiovascular Society includes among its recommendations some options of management for these patients. Thus, renal function must be checked daily in patients with heart failure and increasing serum creatinine more than 30% from baseline, and ACEI, ARB, and aldosterone dose should be reduced until renal function stabilizes. In oliguric HF patients treatment with diuretics, ACEI, ARB, or aldosterone should be reviewed daily. Routine use of ACE inhibitors, ARBs or spironolactone in the setting of severe renal dysfunction (serum creatinine levels greater than 250 μmol/L or an increase of more than 50% from baseline) is not routinely recommended [266].

Anemia is a frequent and multifactorial finding in both CKD and CHF. Its prevalence is similar among patients with preserved and depressed LVEF; a pragmatical strategy for anemia correction has been proposed [267] from many International and National Societies, suggesting an incomplete correction with a target hemoglobin of 10–12 g/dL at clinical practice, because of the adverse cardiovascular effects of higher hematocrit in CKD trials, [267 –268].

References

[1] U.S. Renal Data System. USRDS 2000 Annual Data Report.

[2] Foley RN, Parfrey PS, Sarnak MJ "Epidemiology of cardiovascular disease in chronic renal disease. *J. Am. Soc. Nephrol.* 1998; 9 (12 suppl): S16-23.

[3] Levin A, Singer J, Thompson CR et al. "Prevalent left ventricular hypertrophy in predialysis population: identifying opportunities for intervention". *Am. J. Kidney Dis.* 1996; 27(3): 347-354.

[4] Manjunath G, Tighiouart H, Coresh J et al "Level of kidney function as a risk factor for atherosclerotic cardiovascular outcomes in the community" *J. Am. Coll. Cardiol.* 2000; 41(1):47- 55.

[5] Longenecker JC, Coresh J, Powe NR, Levey AS, Fink NE, Martin A, Klag MJ. "Traditional cardiovascular disease risk factors in dialysis patients compared with the general population: the CHOICE Study". *J. Am. Soc. Nephrol.* 2002 Jul;13(7):1918-27.

[6] Uhlig K, Levey AS, Sarnak MJ "Traditional cardiac risk factors in individuals with chronic kidney disease". *Semin Dial.* 2003 Mar-Apr;16(2):118-27. Review.

[7] Davenport A "Using dialysis machine technology to reduce intradialytic hypotension". *Hemodial Int.* 2011 Oct;15 Suppl 1:S37-42.

[8] Tonelli M, Bohm C, Pandeya S, Gill J, Levin A, Kiberd BA "Cardiac risk factors and the use of cardioprotective medications in patients with chronic renal insufficiency". *Am. J. Kidney Dis.* 2001 Mar;37(3):484-9.

[9] Di Lullo L, Addesse R, Comegna C, Firmi G, Galderisi C, Iannacci GR, Polito P "Effects of fluvastatin treatment on lipid profile, C-reactive protein trend, and renal function in dyslipidemic patients with chronic renal failure". *Adv. Ther.* 2005 Nov-Dec;22(6):601-12.

[10] National Kidney Foundation. K/DOQI Clinical Practice Guidelines for Managing Dyslipidemia in Chronic Kidney Disease. *Am. J. Kidney Dis.* 2003; 41(suppl 3): S1-92.

[11] Herzog CA, Ma JZ, Collins AJ "Comparative survival of dialysis patients in the United States after coronary angioplasty, coronary artery stenting, and coronary artery bypass surgery and impact of diabetes". *Circulation.* 2002 Oct 22;106(17):2207-11.

[12] Blacher J, Pannier B, Guerin AP et al "Carotid arterial stiffness as a predictor of cardiovascular and all-cause mortality in end-stage renal disease". *Hypertension* 1998; 32 (3): 570-574.

[13] Levin A, Thompson CR, Ethier J et al "Left ventricular mass index increase in early renal disease: impact of decline in hemoglobin" *Am. J. Kidney Dis.* 1999; 34(1): 125-134.

[14] Middleton RJ, Parfrey PS, Foley RN "Left ventricular hypertrophy in the renal patient" *J. Am. Soc. Nephrol.* 2001;12 (5): 1079-1084.

[15] Bostom AG, Lathrop L "Hyperhomocysteinemia in end-stage renal disease: prevalence, etiology and potential relationship to arteriosclerotic outcomes. *Kidney Int.* 1997; 52(1): 10-20.

[16] Himmelfarb J, Stenvinkel P, Ikizler TA, Hakim RM "The elephant in uremia: oxidant stress as a unifying concept of cardiovascular disease in uremia" *Kidney Int.* 2002; 62 (5): 1524-1538.

[17] Spittle MA, Hoenich NA, Handelman GJ et al "Oxidative stress and inflammation in hemodialysis patients" *Am. J. Kidney Dis.* 2001; 38 (6): 1408-1413.

[18] Levin A, Thompson CR, Ethier J, "Left ventricular mass index increase in early renal disease: impact in decline of hemoglobin". *Am. J. Kidney Disease* 34(1): 125 – 134, 1999.

[19] Foley RN, Parfrey PS, Kent GM et al "Long-term evolution of cardiomyopathy in dialysis patients". *Kidney Int.* 54 – 1720 – 25, 1998.

[20] Foley RN, Parfrey PS, Harnett JD et al "Clinical and echocardiographic disease in patients starting end – stage renal disease therapy" *Kidney Int.* 47 (1): 186 – 192, 1995.

[21] Tsioufis C, Kokkinos P, Macmanus C, Thomopoulos C, Faselis C, Doumas M, Stefanadis C, Papademetriou V. "Left ventricular hypertrophy as a determinant of renal outcome in patients with high cardiovascular risk "*J. Hypertens.* 2010 Nov; 28(11):2299-308.

[22] Mimura I, Nishi H, Mise N, Mori M, Sugimoto T. "Left ventricular geometry and cardiovascular mortality based on haemodialysis patient autopsy analyses". *Nephrology* (Carlton). 2010 Aug;15(5):549-54.

[23] Dzau VJ "The role of mechanical and humoral factors in growth regulation of vascular smooth muscle and cardiac myocytes". *Curr. Opin. Nephrol. Hypertens* 2(1): 27 – 32, 1993.

[24] Foley RN, Curtis BM, Randell EW, Parfrey PS. "Left ventricular hypertrophy in new hemodialysis patients without symptomatic cardiac disease". *Clin. J. Am. Soc. Nephrol.* 2010 May;5(5):805-13. Epub 2010 Apr 8.

[25] Dimitrijevic Z, Cvetkovic T, Stojanovic M, Paunovic K, Djordjevic V. "Prevalence and risk factors of myocardial remodeling in hemodialysis patients". *Ren. Fail.* 2009;31(8):662-7.

[26] Costa Fde A, Rivera IR, Vasconcelos ML, Costa AF, Póvoa RM, Bombig MT, Luna Filho B, Lima VC. "Electrocardiography in the diagnosis of ventricular hypertrophy in patients with chronic renal disease ". *Arq. Bras. Cardiol.* 2009 Oct;93(4):380-6, 373-9. English, Portuguese, Spanish.

[27] Aoki J, Ikari Y, Nakajima H et al. "Clinical and pathological characteristics of dilated cardiomyopathy in hemodialysis patients" *Kidney Int.* 67: 333 – 340, 2005.

[28] Araujo S, Lemes HP, Cunha DA, Queiroz VS, Nascimento DD, Ferreira Filho SR. "Cardiac morphology and function in patients with and without residual diuresis on hemodialysis". *J. Bras. Nefrol.* 2011 Mar;33(1):74-81. English, Portuguese.

[29] Falcão-Pires I, Leite-Moreira AF. "Diabetic cardiomyopathy: understanding the molecular and cellular basis to progress in diagnosis and treatment". *Heart Fail Rev.* 2011 May 28.

[30] Demers C, Rouleau JL, Leung TK, Tardif JC. "Hypercalcemic cardiomyopathy associated with primary hyperparathyroidism mimicking primary obstructive hypertrophic cardiomyopathy". *Can. J. Cardiol.* 1998 Nov;14(11):1397-400.

[31] Keller E, Moravec CS, Bond M: "Altered subcellular Ca regulation in papillary muscles from cardiomyopathic hearts". *Am. J. Physiol.* 268 (5 pt 2): H1875 – H1883, 1995.

[32] Raizada V, Skipper B, Taylor RA, Luo W, Harford AA, Zager PG, Rohrscheib M, Spalding CT. "Left ventricular diastolic function in patients on hemodialysis". *J. Investig Med.* 2010 Aug;58(6):791-5.

[33] Losi MA, Memoli B, Contaldi C, Barbati G, Del Prete M, Betocchi S, Cavallaro M, Carpinella G, Fundaliotis A, Parrella LS, Parisi V, Guida B, Chiariello M. "Myocardial fibrosis and diastolic dysfunction in patients on chronic haemodialysis". *Nephrol Dial Transplant.* 2010 Jun;25(6):1950-4.

[34] Parfrey PS, Foley RN, Harnett JD et al "Outcome and risk factors for left ventricular disorders in chronic uraemia" *Nephrol Dial Transplant.* 16 (7): 1277 – 1285, 1996.

[35] Goh CY, Vizzi G, De Cal M, Ronco C. "Cardiorenal syndrome: a complex series of combined heart/kidney disorders". *Contrib. Nephrol.* 2011;174:33-45.

[36] Foley RN, Parfrey PS, Kent GM et al "Serial change in echocardiographic parameters and cardiac failure in end – stage renal disease" *J. Am. Soc. Nephrol.* 11:912 – 916, 2000.

[37] Periyasamy SM, Chen J, Cooney D, Carter P, Omran E, Tian J, Priyadarshi S, Bagrov A, Fedorova O, Malhotra D, Xie Z, Shapiro JI. "Effects of uremic serum on isolated cardiac myocyte calcium cycling and contractile function".

[38] Yigla M, Nakhoul F, Sabag A, Tov N, Gorevich B, Abassi Z, Reisner SA. Pulmonary hypertension in patients with end-stage renal disease. *Chest.* 2003.May;123(5):1577-82.

[39] Di Lullo L, Floccari F, Polito P Right ventricular diastolic function in dialysis patients could be affected by vascular access. *Nephron Clin.* Pract 2011; 118: c258 – c262.

[40] Beigi AA, Sadeghi AM, Khosravi AR, Karami M, Masoudpour H. Effects of the arteriovenous fistula on pulmonary artery pressure and cardiac output in patients with chronic renal failure. *J. Vasc. Access.* 2009 Jul-Sep;10(3):160-6.

[41] Rich S, Seidlitz M, Dodin E et al. The short term effects of digoxin in patients with right ventricular dysfunction from pulmonary hypertension. *Chest* 114:787, 1998.

[42] Sitbon O, Humbert M, Simonneau G Primary pulmonary hypertension: Current therapy. *Prog. Cardiovasc. Disease* 45:115, 2002.

[43] Kiykim AA, Horoz M, Ozcan T, Yildiz I, Sari S, Genctoy G. Pulmonary hypertension in hemodialysis patients without arteriovenous fistula: the effect of dialyzer composition. *Ren. Fail.* 2010; 32 (10): 1148-52.

[44] Barst RJ, Gibbs JS, Ghofrani HA, Hoeper MM, McLaughlin VV, Rubin LJ, Sitbon O, Tapson VF, Galiè N *Update evidence based treatment algorithm in pulmonary arterial hypertension Journal American College of Cardiology* 2009, Jun (30); 54 S 78-84.

[45] Sitbon O, Humbert M, Jaïs X, Ioos V, Hamid AM, Provencher S, Garcia G, Parent F, Hervé P, Simonneau G Long-term response to calcium channel blockers in idiopathic pulmonary arterial hypertension. *Circulation,* 2005 Jun 14; 111 (23): 3105-11.

[46] Sitbon O, Humbert M, Nunes H et al. Long – term intravenous epoprostenol infusion in primary pulmonary hypertension. *J. Am. Coll. Cardiol.* 40:780, 2002.

[47] Benza RL, Rayburn BK, Tallaj JA, Pamboukian SV, Bourge RC. Treprostinil-based therapy in the treatment of moderate-to-severe pulmonary arterial hypertension: long-term efficacy and combination with bosentan. *Chest* 2008, Jul; 134 (1): 139-45.

[48] Olschewski H, Simonneau G, Galiè N, Higenbottam T, Naeije R, Rubin LJ et al Inhaled iloprost for severe pulmonary hypertension. *N. Eng. J. Med.* 2002, Aug 1; 347 (5): 322-9.

[49] Galiè N, Humbert M, Vachiéry JL, Vizza CD, Kneussl M, Manes A, Sitbon O, Torbicki A, Delcroix M, Naeije R, Hoeper M, Chaouat A, Morand S, Besse B, Simonneau G; Effects of beraprost sodium, an oral prostacyclin analogue, in patients with pulmonary arterial hypertension: a randomized, double-blind, placebo-controlled trial. *J. Am. Coll. Card.* 2002 May 1; 39 (9): 1496-502.

[50] Galiè N., Rubin L. J., Hoeper M., Jansa P., Al-Hiti H., Meyer G. M. B., Chiossi E., Kusic-Pajic A., Simonneau G. (2008a). Treatment of patients with mildly symptomatic pulmonary arterial hypertension with bosentan (EARLY study): a double-blind, randomised controlled trial. *Lancet* 371, 2093–2100.

[51] Ghofrani H. A., Wiedemann R., Rose F., Schermuly R. T., Olschewski H., Weissmann N., Gunther A., Walmrath D., Seeger W., Grimminger F. (2002b). Sildenafil for treatment of lung fibrosis and pulmonary hypertension: a randomised controlled trial. *Lancet* 360, 895–900.

[52] Yigla M, Abassi Z, Reisner SA, Nakhoul F. Pulmonary hypertension in hemodialysis patients: an unrecognized threat. *Semin Dial.* 2006 Sep-Oct;19(5):353-7.

[53] Abdelwhab S, Elshinnawy S. Pulmonary hypertension in chronic renal failure patients. *Am. J. Nephrol.* 2008;28(6):990-7.

[54] Yigla M, Fruchter O, Ahronson D, Yanay N, Reisner SA, Lewin M, Nakhoul F "Pulmonary hypertension i san independent predictor of mortality in hemodialysis patients – *Kidney Int.* 2009 May, 75(9): 969-75.

[55] Fruchter O, Yigla M "Predictors of long-term survival in elderly patients hospitalized for acute exacerbation of chronic obstructive pulmonary disease" – *Respirology*, 2008 Nov; 13(6):851-5.

[56] Abassi Z, Nakhoul F, Khankin E, Reisner SA, Yigla M. Pulmonary hypertension in chronic dialysis patients with arteriovenous fistula: pathogenesis andtherapeutic prospective. *Curr. Opin. Nephrol. Hypertens.* 2006 Jul;15(4):353-60.

[57] Beigi AA, Sadeghi AM, Khosravi AR, Karami M, Masoudpour H. Effects of the arteriovenous fistula on pulmonary artery pressure and cardiac output in patients with chronic renal failure. *J. Vasc. Access.* 2009 Jul-Sep;10(3):160-6.

[58] Di Lullo L, Floccari F, Granata A, Fiorini F, D'Amelio A, Gorini A, Malaguti M, Polito P. Ecocardiografia e funzione ventricolare destra in pazienti affetti da IRC in stadio III NKF. Congresso Nazionale di Nefrologia, Genova, 21-24 Settembre 2011. *Giornale Italiano di Nefrologia*, 2011, 28, S53, S60.

[59] Gabella G: "*The Pericardium in Gray's Anatomy: The Anatomical Basis of Medicine and Surgery",* 1995 pp 1471 – 72.

[60] Rostand SG, Rutsky EA: "Pericarditis in end-stage renal disease". *Cardiol. Clin.* 8:701, 1998.

[61] Goland S, Caspi A, Malnick S, et al: "Idiopathic chronic pericardial effusion". *N. Eng. J. Med.* 342: 1449, 2000.

[62] LeWinter M, Kabbani S: "Pericardial disease in Braunwald's Heart Disease 7th Ed", 2005.

[63] Otto C. "Textbook of Clinical Echocardiography", 4th Ed, 2009.

[64] Sparano DM, Ward RP "Pericarditis and pericardial effusion: management update". *Curr. Treat Options Cardiovasc. Med.* 2011 Dec;13(6):543-55.

[65] Tseng JR, Lee MJ, Yen KC, Weng CH, Liang CC, Wang IK, Chang CT, Lin-Tan DT, Lin JL, Yen TH. "Course and outcome of dialysis pericarditis in diabetic patients treated with maintenance hemodialysis". *Kidney Blood Press Res.* 2009;32(1):17-23. Epub 2009 Feb 12.

[66] Kudo Y, Yamasaki F, Doi Y, Sugiura T. "Clinical correlates of PR-segment depression in asymptomatic patients with pericardial effusion". *J. Am. Coll. Cardiol.* 2002 Jun 19;39(12):2000-4.

[67] Brandt RR, Filzmaier K, Hanrath P. "Circulating cardiac troponin I in acute pericarditis" *Am. J. Cardiol.* 2001 Jun 1; 87 (11): 1326 – 8.

[68] Imazio M, Brucato A, Mayosi BM, Derosa FG, Lestuzzi C, Macor A, Trinchero R, Spodick DH, Adler Y. "Medical therapy of pericardial diseases: part I: idiopathic and infectious pericarditis". *J. Cardiovasc. Med.* (Hagerstown). 2010 Oct;11(10):712-22. Review.

[69] Zeina AR, Odeh M, Barmeir E. "Chronic constrictive pericarditis". *Clin. Cardiol.* 2010 Aug;33(8):E21.

[70] Khandaker MH, Espinosa RE, Nishimura RA, Sinak LJ, Hayes SN, Melduni RM, Oh JK. "Pericardial disease: diagnosis and management". *Mayo Clin. Proc.* 2010 Jun;85(6):572-93. Review.

[71] U.S. Renal Data System. USRDS 2006 Annual Data Report. National Institutes of Health, National Institute of Diabetes and Digestive and Kidney Diseases, Bethesda, MD, 2006.

[72] Foley, RN, Parfrey, PS, Sarnak, MJ: Clinical epidemiology of cardiovascular disease in chronic renal disease. *Am. J. Kidney Dis.* 1998 32: S112–119.

[73] K/DOQI clinical practiceguidelines for cardiovascular disease in dialysis patients. *Am. J. Kidney Dis.* 2005; 45 /supple 3): S1-153.

[74] Muntner P, Hamm LL, Kusek JW, Chen J, Whelton PK, He J. The prevalence of nontraditional risk factors for coronary heart disease in patients with chronic kidney disease. *Ann. Intern. Med.* 2004; 140:9-17.

[75] Longenecker JC, Coresh J, Powe NR, Levey AS, Fink NE, Martin A, Klag MJ. Traditional ardiovascular disease risk factors in dialysis patients compared with the general population: the CHOICE Study. *J. Am. Soc. Nephrol.* 2002; 13:1918-1927.

[76] Sarnak MJ, Levey AS, Schoolwerth AC, Coresh J, Culleton B, Hamm LL, McCullough PA, Kasiske BL, Kelepouris E, Klag MJ, Parfrey P, Pfeffer M, Raij L, Spinosa DJ, Wilson PW; American Heart Association Councils on Kidney in Cardiovascular Disease, High Blood Pressure Research, Clinical Cardiology, and Epidemiology and Prevention. Kidney disease as a risk factor for development of cardiovascular disease: a statement from the American Heart Association Councils on Kidney in Cardiovascular Disease, High Blood Pressure Research, Clinical Cardiology, and Epidemiology and Prevention. *Circulation.* 2003; 108:2154-2169.

[77] Chertow GM, Normand SL, Silva LR, McNeil BJ. Survival after acute myocardial infarction in patients with end-stage renal disease: results from the cooperative cardiovascular project. *Am. J. Kidney Dis.* 2000; 35:1044-1051.

[78] Hemmelgarn BR, Southern D, Culleton BF, Mitchell LB, Knudtson ML, Ghali WA; Alberta Provincial Project for Outcomes Assessment in Coronary Heart Disease (APPROACH) Investigators. Survival after coronary revascularization among patients with kidney disease. *Circulation.* 2004; 110:1890-1895.

[79] Komukai K, Ogawa T, Yagi H, Date T, Suzuki K, Sakamoto H, Miyazaki H, Takatsuka H, Shibayama K, Ogawa K, Kanzaki Y, Kosuga T, Kawai M, Hongo K, Yoshida S, Taniguchi I, Mochizuki S. Renal insufficiency is related to painless myocardial infarction. *Circ. J.* 2007; 71:1366– 1369.

[80] De Lima JJ, Sabbaga E, Vieira ML, de Paula FJ, Ianhez LE, Krieger EM, Ramires JA. Coronary angiography is the best predictor of events in renal transplant candidates compared with noninvasive testing. *Hypertension.* 2003; 42:263-268.

[81] Marwick TH, Steinmuller DR, Underwood DA, Hobbs RE, Go RT, Swift C, Braun WE. Ineffectiveness of dipyridamole SPECT thallium imaging as a screening technique for coronary artery disease in patients with end-stage renal failure. *Transplantation.* 1990; 49:100-103.

[82] Reis G, Marcovitz PA, Leichtman AB, Merion RM, Fay WP, Werns SW, Armstrong WF. Usefulness of dobutamine stress echocardiography in detecting coronary artery disease in end-stage renal disease. *Am. J. Cardiol.* 1995; 75:707–710.

[83] Herzog CA, Marwich TH, Pheley AM, White CW, Venkateswara KR, Candace DD. Dobutamine stress echocardiography for the detection of significant coronary artery disease in renal transplant candidates. *Am. J. Kidney Dis.* 1999; 33:1080– 1090.

[84] Bates JR, Sawada SG, Segar DS, Spaedy AJ, Petrovic O, Fineberg NS, Ryan T. Evaluation using dobutamine stress echocardiography in patients with insulin-dependent diabetes mellitus before kidney and/or pancreas transplantation. *Am. J. Cardiol.* 1996; 77:175– 179.

[85] Brennan DC, Vedala G, Miller SB, Anstey ME, Singer GG, Kovacs A, Barzilai B, Lowell JA, Shenoy S, Howard TK, Davila-Roman VG. Pretransplant dobutamine stress echocardiography is useful and cost-effective in renal transplant candidates. *Transplant Proc.* 1997; 29: 233–234.

[86] West JC, Napoliello DA, Costello JM, Nassef LA, Butcher RJ, Hartle JE, McConnell TR, Finley JW, Kelley SE, Chao S, Latsha R. Preoperative dobutamine stress echocardiography versus cardiac arteriography for risk assessment prior to renal transplantation. *Transpl. Int.* 2000;13:S27–S30.

[87] Picano E. Dobutamine stress echocardiography. In: Picano E, editor. Stress echocardiography. 4th ed. *Heidelberg Springer-Verlag*;. 2003, pp 115–132.

[88] Pingitore A, Picano E, Varga A, Gigli G, Cortigiani L, Previtali M, Minardi G, Colosso MQ, Lowenstein J, Mathias W Jr, Landi P. Prognostic value of pharmacological stress echocardiography in patients with known or suspected coronary artery disease: a prospective, large scale, multicenter, head-to-head comparison between dipyridamole and do0butamine test. *J. Am. Coll. Cardiol.* 1999; 34:1769–1777.

[89] Rabbat CG, Treleaven DJ, Russell JD, Ludwin D, Cook DJ. Prognostic value of myocardial perfusion studies in patients with end-stage renal disease assessed for kidney or kidney-pancreas transplantation: a meta-analysis. *J. Am. Soc. Nephrol.* 2003 Feb;14(2):431–439.

[90] Fleg JL. Myocardial Ischemia in the Asymptomatic Older Patient. *Am. J. Geriatr. Cardiol.* 1998; 7:54-59.

[91] Faglia E, Favales F, Calia P, Paleari F, Segalini G, Gamba PL, Rocca A, Musacchio N, Mastropasqua A, Testori G, Rampini P, Moratti F, Braga A, Morabito A; Milan Study on Atherosclerosis and Diabetes (Mi SAD). Cardiac events in 735 type 2 diabetic patients who underwent screening for unknown asymptomatic coronary heart disease: 5-year follow-up report from the Milan Study on Atherosclerosis and Diabetes (MiSAD). *Diabetes Care.* 2002; 25:2032-2036.

[92] Janand-Delenne B, Savin B, Habib G, Bory M, Vague P, Lassmann-Vague V. Silent myocardial ischemia in patients with diabetes: who to screen. *Diabetes Care.* 1999; 22:1396-1400.

[93] Gottlieb SO, Weisfeldt ML, Ouyang P, Mellits ED, Gerstenblith G. Silent ischemia as a marker for early unfavorable outcomes in patients with unstable angina. *N. Engl. J. Med.* 1986; 314:1214-1219.

[94] Bennett WM, Kloster F, Rosch J, Barry J, Porter GA. Natural history of asymptomatic coronary arteriographic lesions in diabetic patients with end-stage renal disease. *Am. J Med.* 1978; 65:779-784.

[95] Rivera RF, Mircoli L, Bonforte G, et al. Dipyridamole stress echocardiography in diagnosis and prognosis of hemodialysis patients with asymptomatic coronary disease. *Hemodial Int.* 2011;15(4):468-76.

[96] Rao M, Jaber BL, Balakrishnan VS. Inflammatory biomarkers and cardiovascular risk: association or cause and effect? *Semin Dial.* 2006 Mar-Apr;19(2):129-35.

[97] Chaykovska L, Tsuprykov O, Hocher B. Biomarkers for the prediction of mortality and morbidity in patients with renal replacement therapy. *Clin. Lab.* 2011;57(7-8):455-67.

[98] Watnick S, Perazella MA. Cardiac troponins: utility in renal insufficiency and end-stage renal disease. *Semin Dial.* 2002 Jan-Feb;15(1):66-70.

[99] Ketteler M, Bongartz P, Westenfeld R, et al, 2003 Association of low fetuin-A (AHSG) concentrations in serum with cardiovascular mortality in patients on dialysis: a cross-sectional study. *Lance*t 361: 827–833.

[100] Jüppner H. Phosphate and FGF-23. *Kidney Int. Suppl.* 2011 Apr;(121):S24-7. Epub 2011 Feb 23.

[101] Carrero JJ, Cordeiro AC, Lindholm B, Stenvinkel P. The emerging pleiotrophic role of adipokines in the uremic phenotype. *Curr. Opin. Nephrol. Hypertens.* 2010 Jan;19(1):37-42.

[102] Agaewal, R, Nissenson, AR, Batlle, D, et al: Prevalence, treatment, and control of hypertension in chronic hemodialysis patients in the United States. *Am. J. Med.* 2003 115: 291–297.

[103] Chobanian AV, Bakris GL, Black HR, et al. The Seventh Report of the Joint National Committee on Prevention, Detection, Evaluation, and Treatment of High Blood Pressure: the JNC 7 report. *JAMA* 2003;289:2560–72.

[104] McCullough, PA, Sandberg, KR, Borzak, S, et al: Benefits of aspirin and beta-blockade after myocardial infarction in patients with chronic kidney disease. *Am. Heart J.* 2002 144: 226–232.

[105] Lynn KL. Hypertension and survival in hemodialysis patients. *Semin Dial.* 2004;17:270–4.

[106] Fabbian F, De Giorgi A, Pala M, Tiseo R, Manfredini R, Portaluppi F. Evidence-based statin prescription for cardiovascular protection in renal impairment. *Clin. Exp. Nephrol.* 2011;15(4):456-63.

[107] Di Lullo L, Addesse R, Comegna C, Firmi G, Galderisi C, Iannacci GR, Polito P Effects of fluvastatin therapy on lipid profile, C – reactive protein trend and renal function in dyslipidemic patients with chronic renal failure. *Adv. Ther.* 2005 Nov – Dec; 22(6): 601 – 12.

[108] American Diabetes Association: Standards of medical care for patients with diabetes mellitus. *Diabetes Care* 2003 26(Suppl 1):S33–50.

[109] Winchester, JF. Therapeutic uses of aspirin in renal diseases. *Am. J. Kidney Dis.* 1996 28(Suppl 1):S20–23.

[110] Holzmann MJ, Ahnve S, Hammar N, Jorgensen L, Klerdal K, Pehrsson K, Ivert T. Creatinine clearance and risk of early mortality in patients undergoing coronary artery bypass grafting. *J. Thorac. Cardiovasc. Surg.* 2005;130(3):746–52.

[111] Noyez L, Plesiewicz I, Verheugt FW. Estimated creatinine clearance instead of plasma creatinine level as prognostic test for postoperative renal function in patients undergoing coronary artery bypass surgery. *Eur. J. Cardiothorac. Surg.* 2006;29 (4):461–5.

[112] Cooper WA, O'Brien SM, Thourani VH, Guyton RA, Bridges CR, Szczech LA, et al. Impact of renal dysfunction on outcomes of coronary artery bypass surgery: results from the Society of Thoracic Surgeons National Adult Cardiac Database. *Circulation* 2006;113(8):1063–70.

[113] Best PJ, Lennon R, Ting HH, Bell MR, Rihal CS, Holmes DR, Berger PB. The impact of renal insufficiency on clinical outcomes in patients undergoing percutaneous coronary interventions. *J. Am. Coll. Cardiol.* 2002;39(7):1113–9.

[114] Scolari F, Ravani P, Gaggi R, Santostefano M, Rollino C, Stabellini N, et al. The challenge of diagnosing atheroembolic renal disease: clinical features and prognostic factors. *Circulation* 2007;116(3): 298–304.

[115] Gurm HS, Lincoff AM, Kleiman NS, Kereiakes DJ, Tcheng JE, Aronow HD, et al. Double jeopardy of renal insufficiency and anemia in patients undergoing percutaneous coronary interventions. *Am. J. Cardiol.* 2004;94(1):30–4.

[116] Pinkau T, Hilgers KF, Veelken R, Mann JF. How does minor renal dysfunction influence cardiovascular risk and the management of cardiovascular disease? *J. Am. Soc. Nephrol.* 2004; 15(3):517–23.

[117] Rinehart AL, Herzog CA, Collins AJ, Flack JM, Ma JZ, Opsahl JA. A comparison of coronary angioplasty and coronary artery bypass grafting outcomes in chronic dialysis patients. *Am. J. Kidney Dis.* 1995;25(2):281–90.

[118] Reddan DN, Szczech LA, Tuttle RH, Shaw LK, Jones RH, Schwab SJ, et al. Chronic kidney disease, mortality, and treatment strategies among patients with clinically significant coronary artery disease. *J. Am. Soc. Nephrol.* 2003;14(9):2373–80.

[119] Ivens K, Gradaus F, Heering P, Schoebel FC, Klein M, Schulte HD, et al. Myocardial revascularization in patients with end-stage renal disease: comparison of percutaneous transluminal coronary angioplasty and coronary artery bypass grafting. *Int. Urol. Nephrol.* 2001;32(4):717–23.

[120] Aoki J, Ong AT, Hoye A, van Herwerden LA, Sousa JE, Jatene A, et al. Five year clinical effect of coronary stenting and coronary artery bypass grafting in renal insufficient patients with multivessel coronary artery disease: insights from ARTS trial. *Eur. Heart J.* 2005;26(15):1488–93.

[121] Halkin A, Mehran R, Casey CW, Gordon P, Matthews R, Wilson BH, et al. Impact of moderate renal insufficiency on restenosis and adverse clinical events after paclitaxel-eluting and bare metal stent implantation: results from the TAXUS-IV Trial. *Am. Heart J.* 2005;150(6):1163–70.

[122] Herzog CA, Ma JZ, Collins AJ. Comparative survival of dialysis patients in the United States after coronary angioplasty, coronary artery stenting, and coronary artery bypass surgery and impact of diabetes. *Circulation* 2002;106(17):2207–11.

[123] Herzog CA, Ma JZ, Collins AJ. Long-term outcome of dialysis patients in the United States with coronary revascularization procedures. *Kidney Int.* 1999;56(1):324–32.

[124] Das P, Moliterno DJ, Charnigo R, Mukherjee D, Steinhubl SR, Sneed JD, et al. Impact of drug-eluting stents on outcomes of patients with end-stage renal disease undergoing percutaneous coronary revascularization. *J. Invasive Cardiol.* 2006;18 (9):405–8.

[125] Levey AS, Coresh J, Balk E, et al. National Kidney Foundation practice guidelines for chronic kidney disease: evaluation, classification, and stratification. *Ann. Intern. Med.* 2003 Jul 15;139(2):137-47.

[126] Obrador GT, Ruthazer R, Arora P, Kausz AT, Pereira BJ. Prevalence of and factors associated with suboptimal care before initiation of dialysis in the United States. *J. Am. Soc. Nephrol.* Aug 1999;10(8): 1793-800.

[127] Centers for Disease Control and Prevention. Prevalence of chronic kidney disease and associated risk factors--United States, 1999-2004. *MMWR Morb. Mortal. Wkly. Rep.* Mar 2 2007;56(8):161-5.

[128] Moranne et al., 2009 O. Moranne, M. Froissart and J. Rossert, et al. Timing of onset of CKD-related metabolic complications. *Journal of the American Society of Nephrology,* 20 (2009), pp. 164–171.

[129] Lea JP, Norris K, Agodoa L. The role of anemia management in improving outcomes for African-Americans with chronic kidney disease. *Am. J. Nephrol.* 2008;28(5): 732–743.

[130] McFarlane SI, Chen SC, Whaley-Connell AT, et al. Prevalence and associations of anemia of CKD: Kidney Early Evaluation Program (KEEP) and National Health and Nutrition Examination Survey (NHANES) 1999–2004. *Am. J. Kidney Dis.* 2008;51(4 Suppl 2):S46–55.

[131] Caro J, Erslev AJ. Uremic inhibitors of erythropoiesis. *Semin Nephrol.* 1985;5: 128-132.

[132] KDOQI Clinical Practice Guideline and Clinical Practice Recommendations for Anemia in Chronic Kidney Disease, 2007 Update of Hemoglobin Target. *Am. J. Kidney Dis.*, September 2007 supplement.

[133] Pfeffer MA, Burdmann EA, Chen CY, et al. A trial of darbepoetin alfa in type 2 diabetes and chronic kidney disease. *N. Engl. J. Med.* 2009; 361: 2019-32.

[134] Singh AK. ESAs in dialysis patients: are you a hedgehog or a fox? *J. Am. Soc. Nephrol.* 2010; 21 (4):543-6.

[135] Radtke HW, Rege AB, Lamarche B, Bartos D, Bartos F, Cambell RA, Fisher JW. Identification of spermine as an inhibitor of erythropoiesis in patients with chronic renal failure. *J. Clin. Invest.* 1981; 67: 1623-1629.

[136] Massry SG. Is parathyroid hormone an uremic toxin? *Nephron* 1977; 19: 125-130.

[137] Stenvinkel P, Heimburger O, Paultre F et al. Strong association between malnutrition, inflammation and atherosclerosis in chronic renal failure. *Kidney Int.* 1999; 55: 1899-1911.

[138] Jongen-Lavrencic M, Peeters HRM, Rozemuller H et al. IL-6 induced anaemia in rats: possible pathogenetic implications for anaemia observed in chronic inflammations. *Clin. Exp. Immunol.* 1996; 103: 328-334.

[139] Goicoechea M, Martin J, de Sequera P, Quiroga JA, Ortiz A, Carreno V, Caramelo C. Role of cytokines in the response to erythropoietin in haemodialysis patients. *Kidney Int.* 1998; 54: 1337-1343.
[140] Kletzmayr J, Mayer G, Legenstein E, Heinz-Peer G, Leitha T, Horl WH, Kovarik J. Anemia and carnitine supplementation in hemodialyzed patients. *Kidney Int.* 1999; 69 (Suppl): 93-106.
[141] Ferrari P, Mallon D, Trinder D, Olynyk JK. Pentoxifylline improves haemoglobin and interleukin-6 levels in chronic kidney disease. *Nephrology* (Carlton) 2010; 15(3): 344-9.
[142] Gaweda AE, Goldsmith LJ, Brier ME, Aronoff GR. Iron, inflammation, dialysis adequacy, nutritional status, and hyperparathyroidism modify erythropoietic response. *Clin. J. Am. Soc. Nephrol.* 2010; 5(4): 576-81.
[143] Ifudu O, Feldman J, Friedman EA. The intensity of haemodialysis and the response to erythropoietin in patients with end-stage renal disease. *New. Engl. J. Med.* 1996; 334: 420-425.
[144] Shooley JC, Kullgren B, Allison AC. Inhibition by interleukin-1 of the action of erythropoietin on erythroid precursors and its possible role in the pathogenesis of hypoplastic anaemias. *Br. J. Haematol.* 1987; 67: 11-17.
[145] Cooper AC, Mikhail A, Lethbridge MW, Kemeny DM, Macdougall IC: Increased expression of erythropoiesis inhibiting cytokines (IFN-gamma, TNF-alpha, IL-10, and IL-13) by T cells in patients exhibiting a poor response to erythropoietin therapy. *J. Am. Soc. Nephrol.* 2003; 14(7): 1776-84.
[146] Panichi V, Scatena A, Paoletti S, Migliori M. Impact of dialysis technique on renal anemia. *Contrib. Nephrol.* 2011;171:261-5.
[147] Madore F, Lowrie EG, Brugnara C, Lew NL, Lazarus JM, Bridges K, Owen WF. Anemia in haemodialysis patients: variables affecting this outcome predictor. *J. Am. Soc. Nephrol.* 1997; 8: 1921-1929.
[148] Coladonato JA, Frankenfield DL, Reddan DN, Klassen PS, Szczech LA, Johnson CA, Owen WF Jr. Trends in anemia management among US haemodialysis patients. *J. Am. Soc. Nephrol.* 2002; 13: 1288-1295.
[149] Eleftheriadis T, Liakopoulos V, Antoniadi G, Kartsios C, Stefanidis I. The role of hepcidin in iron homeostasis and anemia in hemodialysis patients. *Semin Dial.* 2009 Jan-Feb;22(1):70-7.
[150] Yee J, Zasuwa G, Frinak S, Besarab A. Hemoglobin variability and hyporesponsiveness: much ado about something or nothing?*Adv. Chronic Kidney Dis.* 2009 Mar;16(2):83-93.
[151] Elliott DA. Nutritional considerations for the dialytic patient. *Vet. Clin. North Am. Small Anim. Pract.* 2011 Jan;41(1):239-50.
[152] Gandra SR, Finkelstein FO, Bennett AV, et al. Impact of erythropoiesis-stimulating agents on energy and physical function in nondialysis CKD patients with anemia: a systematic review. *Am. J. Kidney Dis.* 2010;55:519-534.
[153] Wish JB, Coyne DW. Use of erythropoiesis-stimulating agents in patients with anemia of chronic kidney disease: overcoming the pharmacological and pharmacoeconomic limitations of existing therapies. *Mayo Clin. Proc.* 2007;82(11):1371-80.

[154] Besarab A, Coyne DW. Iron supplementation to treat anemia in patients with chronic kidney disease. *Nat. Rev. Nephrol.* 2010 Dec;6(12):699-710.

[155] Nakanishi T, Kuragano T, Nanami M, Otaki Y, Nonoguchi H, Hasuike Y.Importance of ferritin for optimizing anemia therapy in chronic kidney disease. *Am. J. Nephrol.* 2010;32(5):439-46.

[156] United States Renal Data System. Excerpts from USRDS 2009 Annual Data Report. U.S.Department of Health and Human Services. The National Institutes of Health, National Institute of Diabetes and Digestive and Kidney Diseases. *Am. J. Kidney Dis.* 2010;55:S1.

[157] London GM, Guerin AP, Marchais SJ, Metivier F, Pannier B, Adda H. Arterial media calcification in end-stage renal disease: impact on all-cause and cardiovascular mortality. *Nephrol. Dial Transplant.* 2003;18:1731-40.

[158] Blacher J, Guerin AP, Pannier B, Marchais SJ, London GM. Arterial calcifications, arterial stiffness, and cardiovascular risk in end-stage renal disease. *Hypertension.* 2001;38:938-42.

[159] Braun J, Oldendorf M, Moshage W, Heidler R, Zeitler E, Luft FC. Electron beam computed tomography in the evaluation of cardiac calcification in chronic dialysis patients. *Am. J. Kidney Dis.* 1996;27:394-401.

[160] Merjanian R, Budoff M, Adler S, Berman N, Mehrotra R.Coronary artery, aortic wall, and valvular calcification in nondialyzed individuals with type 2 diabetes and renal disease. *Kidney Int.* 2003;64:263-71.

[161] Shanahan CM, Cary NR, Salisbury JR, Proudfoot D, Weissberg PL, Edmonds ME. Medial localization of mineralization-regulating proteins in association with Mönckeberg's sclerosis: evidence for smooth muscle cell-mediated vascular calcification. *Circulation.* 1999;100:2168-76.

[162] Proudfoot D, Davies JD, Skepper JN, Weissberg PL, Shanahan CM. Acetylated low-density lipoprotein stimulates human vascular smooth muscle cell calcification by promoting osteoblastic differentiation and inhibiting phagocytosis. *Circulation.* 2002;106:3044-50.

[163] Giachelli CM. Vascular calcification mechanisms. *J. Am. Soc. Nephrol.* 2004;15:2959-64.

[164] Colinayo VV, Qiao JH, Demant P, Krass K, Lusis AJ, Drake TA. Genetic characterization of the Dyscalc locus. *Mamm Genome*. 2002;13:283-8.

[165] Matsui Y, Rittling SR, Okamoto H, et al. Osteopontin deficiency attenuates atherosclerosis in female apolipoprotein E-deficient mice. *Arterioscler Thromb. Vasc. Biol.* 2003;23:1029-34.

[166] Pan JH, Sukhova GK, Yang JT, et al. Macrophage migration inhibitory factor deficiency impairs atherosclerosis in low-density lipoprotein receptor-deficient mice. *Circulation*. 2004;109:3149-53.

[167] Luo G, Ducy P, McKee MD, et al. Spontaneous calcification of arteries and cartilage in mice lacking matrix GLA protein. *Nature.* 1997;386:78-81.

[168] Speer MY, Chien YC, Quan M, et al. Smooth muscle cells deficient in osteopontin have enhanced susceptibility to calcification in vitro. *Cardiovasc. Res.* 2005;66:324-33.

[169] Kuro-o M, Matsumura Y, Aizawa H, et al. Mutation of the mouse klotho gene leads to a syndrome resembling ageing. *Nature.* 1997;390:45-51.

[170] Spicer SS, Lewis SE, Tashian RE, Schulte BA. Mice carrying a CAR-2 null allele lack carbonic anhydrase II immunohistochemically and show vascular calcification. *Am. J. Pathol.* 1989;134:947-54.

[171] Schafer C, Heiss A, Schwarz A, et al. The serum protein alpha 2-Heremans-Schmid glycoprotein/fetuin-A is a systemically acting inhibitor of ectopic calcification. *J. Clin. Invest.* 2003;112:357-66.

[172] Musunuru K, Post WS, Herzog W, et al. Association of single nucleotide polymorphisms on chromosome 9p21.3 with platelet reactivity: a potential mechanism for increased vascular disease. *Circ. Cardiovasc. Genet.* 2010,3:445-53.

[173] Burdon KP, Rudock ME, Lehtinen AB, et al. Human lipoxygenase pathway gene variation and association with markers of subclinical atherosclerosis in the diabetes heart study. *Mediators Inflamm.*;2010:170153.

[174] Schmitz F, Ewering S, Zerres K, Klomfass S, Hoffmann R, Ortlepp JR. Parathyroid hormone gene variant and calcific aortic stenosis. *J. Heart Valve. Dis.* 2009;18:262-7.

[175] Freedman BI, Bowden DW, Ziegler JT, et al. Bone morphogenetic protein 7 (BMP7) gene polymorphisms are associated with inverse relationships between vascular calcification and BMD: the Diabetes Heart Study. *J. Bone Miner Res.* 2009;24:1719-27.

[176] El-Abbadi MM, Pai AS, Leaf EM, et al. Phosphate feeding induces arterial medial calcification in uremic mice: role of serum phosphorus, fibroblast growth factor-23, and osteopontin. *Kidney Int.* 2009;75: 1297-307.

[177] Goodman WG, Goldin J, Kuizon BD, et al. Coronary-artery calcification in young adults with end-stage renal disease who are undergoing dialysis. *N. Engl. J. Med.* 2000;342:1478-83.

[178] Chertow GM, Raggi P, Chasan-Taber S, Bommer J, Holzer H, Burke SK. Determinants of progressive vascular calcification in haemodialysis patients. *Nephrol. Dial Transplant.* 2004;19:1489-96.

[179] Phan O, Ivanovski O, Nikolov IG, et al. Effect of oral calcium carbonate on aortic calcification in apolipoprotein E-deficient (apoE-/-) mice with chronic renal failure. *Nephrol. Dial Transplant.* 2008;23: 82-90.

[180] Ossareh S, Alaei A, Saedi D. Carotid intima-media thickness in maintenance hemodialysis patients: role of cardiovascular risk factor. *Iran. J. Kidney Dis.* 2011;5: 169-74.

[181] Block GA, Spiegel DM, Ehrlich J, et al. Effects of sevelamer and calcium on coronary artery calcification in patients new to hemodialysis. *Kidney Int.* 2005;68: 1815-24.

[182] Mathew S, Lund RJ, Strebeck F, Tustison KS, Geurs T, Hruska KA. Reversal of the adynamic bone disorder and decreased vascular calcification in chronic kidney disease by sevelamer carbonate therapy. *J. Am. Soc. Nephrol.* 2007;18:122-30.

[183] Yang H, Curinga G, Giachelli CM. Elevated extracellular calcium levels induce smooth muscle cell matrix mineralization in vitro. *Kidney Int.* 2004;66:2293-9.

[184] Adragao T, Pires A, Lucas C, et al. A simple vascular calcification score predicts cardiovascular risk in haemodialysis patients. *Nephrol. Dial Transplant*. 2004;19: 1480-8.

[185] Oh J, Wunsch R, Turzer M, et al. Advanced coronary and carotid arteriopathy in young adults with childhood-onset chronic renal failure. *Circulation*. 2002;106:100-5.

[186] Goldsmith DJ, Covic A, Sambrook PA, Ackrill P. Vascular calcification in long-term haemodialysis patients in a single unit: a retrospective analysis. *Nephron*. 1997; 77:37-43.

[187] Shao JS, Cheng SL, Charlton-Kachigian N, Loewy AP, Towler DA. Teriparatide (human parathyroid hormone (1-34)) inhibits osteogenic vascular calcification in diabetic low density lipoprotein receptor-deficient mice. *J. Biol. Chem.* 2003;278:50195-202.

[188] Zehnder D, Bland R, Chana RS, et al. Synthesis of 1,25-dihydroxyvitamin D(3) by human endothelial cells is regulated by inflammatory cytokines: a novel autocrine determinant of vascular cell adhesion. *Am. Soc. Nephrol*. 2002;13:621-9.

[189] Watson KE, Abrolat ML, Malone LL, et al. Active serum vitamin D levels are inversely correlated with coronary calcification. *Circulation*. 1997;96:1755-60.

[190] Braam LA, Hoeks AP, Brouns F, Hamulyák K, Gerichhausen MJ, Vermeer C. Beneficial effects of vitamins D and K on the elastic properties of the vessel wall in postmenopausal women: a follow-up study. *Thromb. Haemost*. 2004;91:373-80.

[191] Briese S, Wiesner S, Will JC, et al. Arterial and cardiac disease in young adults with childhood-onset end-stage renal disease-impact of calcium and vitamin D therapy. *Nephrol. Dial Transplant*. 2006;21:1906-14.

[192] McCullough PA, Sandberg KR, Dumler F, Yanez JE. Determinants of coronary vascular calcification in patients with chronic kidney disease and end-stage renal disease: a systematic review. *Nephrol*. 2004 Mar-;17:205-15.

[193] Memon F, El-Abbadi M, Nakatani T, Taguchi T, Lanske B, Razzaque MS. Does Fgf23-klotho activity influence vascular and soft tissue calcification through regulating mineral ion metabolism? *Kidney Int*. 2008;74:566-70.

[194] Iyemere VP, Proudfoot D, Weissberg PL, Shanahan CM. Vascular smooth muscle cell phenotypic plasticity and the regulation of vascular calcification. *J. Intern. Med.* 2006;260:192-210.

[195] Anderson HC. Molecular biology of matrix vesicles. *Clin. Orthop. Relat. Res.* 1995;:266-80.

[196] Kim KM. Calcification of matrix vesicles in human aortic valve and aortic media. *Fed. Proc*. 1976;35:156-62.

[197] Reynolds JL, Joannides AJ, Skepper JN, et al. Human vascular smooth muscle cells undergo vesicle-mediated calcification in response to changes in extracellular calcium and phosphate concentrations: a potential mechanism for accelerated vascular calcification in ESRD. *J. Am. Soc. Nephrol*. 2004;15:2857-67.

[198] Littlewood TD, Bennett MR. Apoptotic cell death in atherosclerosis. *Curr. Opin. Lipidol*. 2003;14:469-75.

[199] Kim HH, Kim K. Enhancement of TNF-alpha-mediated cell death in vascular smooth muscle cells through cytochrome c-independent pathway by the proteasome inhibitor. *FEBS Lett*. 2003;535:190-4.

[200] Wada T, McKee MD, Steitz S, Giachelli CM. Calcification of vascular smooth muscle cell cultures: inhibition by osteopontin. *Circ. Res*. 1999;84:166-78.

[201] Ketteler M, Bongartz P, Westenfeld R, et al. Association of low fetuin-A (AHSG) concentrations in serum with cardiovascular mortality in patients on dialysis: a cross-sectional study. *Lancet*. 2003;361:827-33.

[202] Stenvinkel P, Wang K, Qureshi AR, et al. Low fetuin-A levels are associated with cardiovascular death: Impact of variations in the gene encoding fetuin. *Kidney Int*. 2005;67:2383-92.

[203] Price PA, June HH, Buckley JR, Williamson MK. Osteoprotegerin inhibits artery calcification induced by warfarin and by vitamin D. *Arterioscler Thromb. Vasc. Biol*. 2001;21:1610-6.

[204] Rennenberg RJ, Kessels AG, Schurgers LJ, van Engelshoven JM, de Leeuw PW, Kroon AA. Vascular calcifications as a marker of increased cardiovascular risk: a meta-analysis. *Vasc. Health Risk Manag*. 2009;5:185-97.

[205] Blacher J, Safar ME, Pannier B, Guerin AP, Marchais SJ, London GM. Prognostic significance of arterial stiffness measurements in end-stage renal disease patients. *Curr. Opin. Nephrol Hypertens*. 2002;11:629-34.

[206] Guérin AP, Pannier B, Marchais SJ, London GM. Cardiovascular disease in the dialysis population: prognostic significance of arterial disorders. *Curr. Opin. Nephrol Hypertens*. 2006;15:105-10.

[207] London GM. Cardiovascular calcifications in uremic patients: clinical impact on cardiovascular function. *J. Am. Soc. Nephrol*. 2003; 14:S305-9.

[208] Safar ME, Blacher J, Pannier B, et al. Central pulse pressure and mortality in end-stage renal disease. *Hypertension*. 2002;39:735-8.

[209] Kidney Disease: Improving Global Outcomes (KDIGO) CKD-MBD Work Group. KDIGO clinical practice guideline for the diagnosis, evaluation, prevention, and treatment of Chronic Kidney Disease-Mineral and Bone Disorder (CKD-MBD). *Kidney Int. Suppl*. 2009; S1-130.

[210] Tonelli M, Wiebe N, Culleton B, et al; Alberta Kidney Disease Network. Systematic review of the clinical efficacy and safety of sevelamer in dialysis patients. *Nephrol. Dial Transplant*. 2007;22: 2856-66.

[211] Raggi P, Chertow GM, Torres PU, et al; on behalf of the ADVANCE Study Group. The ADVANCE study: a randomized study to evaluate the effects of cinacalcet plus low-dose vitamin D on vascular calcification in patients on hemodialysis. *Nephrol Dial Transplant*. 2011;26:1327-1339.

[212] Clinicaltrials.gov [homepage on the internet] EValuation Of Cinacalcet HCl Therapy to Lower CardioVascular Events. Available from: *http://clinicaltrials.gov/ct2/show/* NCT00345839.

[213] Stenvinkel P: Chronic kidney disease: a public health priority and harbinger of premature cardiovascular disease. *J. Intern. Med*. 2010, 268:456-67.

[214] Carrero JJ, Stenvinkel P: Inflammation in end-stage renal disease–what have we learned in 10 years? *Semin Dial* 2010,23:498-509.

[215] Nathan C, Ding A. Nonresolving inflammation. *Cell* 2010; 140: 871 – 882.

[216] Stassen FR, Vainas T, Bruggeman CA. Infection and atherosclerosis. An alternative view on an outdated hypothesis. *Pharmacol Rep*. 2008; 60: 85 – 92.

[217] Chatzizisis YS, Coskun AU, Jonas M, Edelman ER, Feldman CL, Stone PH. Role of endothelial shear stress in the natural history of coronary atherosclerosis and vascular remodeling: Molecular, cellular, and vascular behavior. *J. Am. Coll. Cardiol.* 2007; 49: 2379 –2393.

[218] Moore Kathryn J, Tabas I. Macrophages in the pathogenesis of atherosclerosis. *Cell* 2011; 145: 341 – 355.

[219] Takeuchi O, Akira S. Pattern recognition receptors and inflammation. *Cell* 2010; 140: 805 – 820.

[220] Rosin DL, Okusa MD. Dangers within: DAMP responses to damage and cell death in kidney disease. *J. Am. Soc. Nephrol.* 2011; 22: 416 –425.

[221] Miller YI, Choi SH, Wiesner P, Fang L, Harkewicz R, Hartvigsen K, et al. Oxidation-specific epitopes are danger-associated molecular patterns recognized by pattern recognition receptors of innate immunity. *Circ. Res*. 2011; 108: 235 – 248.

[222] Seimon TA, Nadolski MJ, Liao X, Magallon J, Nguyen M, Feric NT, et al. Atherogenic lipids and lipoproteins trigger CD36-TLR2-dependent apoptosis in macrophages undergoing endoplasmic reticulum stress. *Cell Metab.* 2010; 12: 467 – 482.

[223] Duewell P, Kono H, Rayner KJ, Sirois CM, Vladimer G, Bauernfeind FG, et al. Nlrp3 inflammasomes are required for atherogenesis and activated by cholesterol crystals. *Nature* 2010; 464: 1357 – 1361.

[224] Suganami T, Ogawa Y. Adipose tissue macrophages: Their role in adipose tissue remodeling. *J. Leukocyte Biol*. 2010; 88: 33 – 39.

[225] Hansson GK, Hermansson A. The immune system in atherosclerosis. *Nat. Immunol.* 2011; 12: 204 – 212.

[226] Nagata S, Hanayama R, Kawane K. Autoimmunity and the clearance of dead cells. *Cell* 2010; 140: 619 – 630.

[227] Baumgarth N. The double life of a B-1 cell: Self-reactivity selects for protective effector functions. *Nat. Rev. Immunol.* 2011; 11: 34 – 46.

[228] Chou MY, Fogelstrand L, Hartvigsen K, Hansen LF, Woelkers D, Shaw PX, et al. Oxidation-specific epitopes are dominant targets of innate natural antibodies in mice and humans. *J. Clin. Invest*. 2009; 119: 1335 – 1349.

[229] Binder CJ, Horkko S, Dewan A, Chang MK, Kieu EP, Goodyear CS, et al. Pneumococcal vaccination decreases atherosclerotic lesion formation: Molecular mimicry between streptococcus pneumoniae and oxidized ldl. *Nat. Med.* 2003; 9: 736 – 743.

[230] Kosteli A, Sugaru E, Haemmerle G, Martin JF, Lei J, Zechner R, et al. Weight loss and lipolysis promote a dynamic immune response in murine adipose tissue. *J. Clin. Invest.* 2010; 120: 3466 – 3479.

[231] Himmelfarb J, Phinney S, Ikizler TA, Kane J, McMonagle E, Miller G: Gamma-tocopherol and docosahexaenoic acid decrease inflammation in dialysis patients. *J. Renal. Nutr.* 2007, 17:296-304.

[232] Fanti P, Asmis R, Stephenson TJ, Sawaya BP, Franke AA. Positive effect of dietary soy in ESRD patients with systemic inflammation - correlation between blood levels of the soy isoflavones and the acute-phase reactants. *Nephrol. Dial Transpl.* 2006, 21:2239-46.

[233] Hsu SP, Wu MS, Yang CC, Huang KC, Liou SY, Hsu SM, Chien CT: Chronic green tea extract supplementation reduces hemodialysis- enhanced production of hydrogen peroxide and hypochlorous acid, atherosclerotic factors, and proinflammatory cytokines. *Am. J. Clin. Nutr.* 2007, 86:1539-47.

[234] Matias PJ, Jorge C, Ferreira C, Borges M, Aires I, Amaral T, Gil C, Cortez J, Ferreira A: Cholecalciferol supplementation in hemodialysis patients: Effects on mineral metabolism, inflammation, and cardiac dimension parameters. *Clin. J. Am. Soc. Nephrol.* 2010, 5:905-11.

[235] Caglar K, Yilmaz MI, Saglam M, Cakir E, Acikel C, Eyileten T, Yenicesu M, Oguz Y, Vural A, Carrero JJ, Axelsson J, Lindholm B, Stenvinkel P: Short-term treatment with sevelamer increases serum fetuin-a concentration and improves endothelial dysfunction in chronic kidney disease stage 4 patients. *Clin. J. Am. Soc. Nephrol.* 2008, 3:61-8.

[236] Fellstrom BC, Jardine AG, Schmieder RE, Holdaas H, Bannister K, Beutler J, Chae DW, Chevaile A, Cobbe SM, Grönhagen-Riska C, De Lima JJ, Lins R, Mayer G, McMahon AW, Parving HH, Remuzzi G, Samuelsson O, Sonkodi S, Sci D, Süleymanlar G, Tsakiris D, Tesar V, Todorov V, Wiecek A, Wüthrich RP, Gottlow M, Johnsson E, Zannad F; AURORA Study Group: Rosuvastatin and cardiovascular events in patients undergoing hemodialysis. *N. Engl. J. Med.* 2009, 360:1395-407.

[237] Goldfine AB, Fonseca V, Jablonski KA, Pyle L, Staten MA, Shoelson SE. The effects of salsalate on glycemic control in patients with type 2 diabetes: A randomized trial. *Ann. Intern. Med.* 2010; 152: 346 –357.

[238] Donath MY, Shoelson SE. Type 2 diabetes as an inflammatory disease. *Nat. Rev. Immunol.* 2011; 11: 98 – 107.

[239] Kleinbongard P, Heusch G, Schulz R. TNFα in atherosclerosis, myocardial ischemia/reperfusion and heart failure. Pharmacol Ther 2010;

[240] 127: 295 – 314.Don BR, Kim K, Li J, Dwyer T, Alexander F, Kaysen GA. The effect of etanercept on suppression of the systemic inflammatory response in chronic hemodialysis patients. *Clin. Nephrol.* 2010,73:431-8.

[241] C. Ronco. The Cardiorenal Syndrome: Basis and Common Ground for a Multidisciplinary Patient-Oriented Therapy. *Cardioren Med.,* 2011;1:3–4.

[242] Goldberg A, Kogan E, Hammerman et al. The impact of transient and persistent acute kidney injury on long-term outcomes in acute myocardial infarction. *Kidney Int.*, 2009, 76(8):900-6.

[243] Mentz RJ, Lewis EF. Epidemiology of cardiorenal syndrome. *Cardiol. Clin.* 2011, 29(2):301-14.

[244] Pannu N, Hemmelgarn B; Alberta Kidney Disease Network. The acute kidney injury to chronic kidney disease continuum: comment on "The magnitude of acute serum

creatinine increase after cardiac surgery and the risk of chronic kidney disease, progression of kidney disease, and death". *Arch. Intern. Med.* 2011 14;171(3):233-4.

[245] Ishani A, Nelson D, Clothier B, Schult T, Nugent S, Greer N, Slinin Y, Ensrud KE. The magnitude of acute serum creatinine increase after cardiac surgery and the risk of chronic kidney disease, progression of kidney disease, and death. *Arch. Intern. Med.* 2011 Feb 14;171(3): 226-33.

[246] McCullough PA, Ahmad A. Cardiorenal syndromes. *World J. Cardiol.* 2011, 26;3(1):1-9.

[247] Go AS, Yang J, Ackerson LM, Lepper K, Robbins S, Massie BM, Shlipak MG. Hemoglobin level, chronic kidney disease, and the risks of death and hospitalization in adults with chronic heart failure: the Anemia in Chronic Heart Failure: Outcomes and Resource Utilization (ANCHOR) Study. *Circulation.* 2006,13;113(23):2713-23.

[248] D. Kennedy, S. Vetteth, M. Sankaridrug et al Central role for the cardiotonic steroid marinobufagenin in the pathogenesis of experimental uremic cardiomiopathy. *Hypertension* 2006;47;488-495.

[249] R. Rabkin,I. Awwad, Y. Chen, et al. Low-Dose Growth Hormone is Cardioprotective in Uremia. *J. Am. Soc. Nephrol.* 19: 1774–1783, 2008.

[250] Aikawa E, Aikawa M, Libby P, et al. Arterial and aortic valve calcification abolished by elastolytic cathepsin S deficiency in chronic renal disease. *Circulation* 2009; 119:1785-1794.

[251] N. Koleganova, G. Piecha, E. Ritz et al. Interstitial fibrosis and microvascular disease of the heart in uremia: amelioration by a calcimimetic. *Lab. Invest.* 2009, 89, 520–530.

[252] Saito Y. Roles of atrial natriuretic peptide and its therapeutic use. J. *Cardiol.* 2010;56(3):262-70.

[253] Kelly KJ. Acute renal failure: much more than a kidney disease. *Semin Nephrol.* 2006; 26(2):105-13.

[254] Casas-Aparicio G, Castillo-Martínez L, Orea-Tejeda A, Abasta-Jiménez M, Keirns-Davies C, Rebollar-González V. The effect of successful kidney transplantation on ventricular dysfunction and pulmonary hypertension. *Transplant Proc.* 2010;42(9):3524-8.

[255] Di Lullo L, Floccari F, Granata A, D'Amelio A, Rivera F, Fiorini F, Malaguti M, Timio M. Ultrasonography: Ariadne's Thread in the Diagnosis of Cardio Renal Syndrome. *Cardiorenal Med.* 2012; 2: 11 – 17.

[256] Licurse A, Kim MC, Dziura J, Forman HP, Formica RN, Makarov DV, Parikh CR, Gross CP. Renal ultrasonography in the evaluation of acute kidney injury: developing a risk stratification framework. *Arch. Intern. Med.* 2010; 22;170(21):1900-7.

[257] Ozmen CA, Akin D, Bilek SU, Bayrak AH, Senturk S, Nazaroglu H. Ultrasound as a diagnostic tool to differentiate acute from chronic renal failure. *Clin. Nephrol.* 2010 Jul;74(1):46-52.

[258] Darmon M, Schortgen F, Vargas F, Liazydi A, Schlemmer B, Brun-Buisson C, Brochard L. Diagnostic accuracy of Doppler renal resistive index for reversibility of acute kidney injury in critically ill patients. *Intensive Care Med.* 2011;37(1):68-76.

[259] Di Lullo L, Floccari F, Granata A, Fiorini F, Polito P. Dyspnea in hemodialysis and early echocardiography examination at the bedside: two case report. *J. Ultrasound.*, 2011, 1-3.

[260] F. Mallamaci, FA. Benedetto, R Tripepi, S Rastelli, P Castellino, G Tripepi, E Picano, C Zoccali, Detection of Pulmonary Congestion by Chest Ultrasound in Dialysis Patients. *J. Am. Coll. Cardiol. Img.* 2010;3:586–94.

[261] Di Lullo L, Floccari F, Polito P Right ventricular diastolic function in dialysis patients could be affected by vascular access. *Nephron. Clin. Pract.* 2011; 118: c258 – c262.

[262] Dickstein K, Cohen-Solal A, Filippatos G, et al. ESC Guidelines for the diagnosis and treatment of acute and chronic heart failure 2008. The Task Force for the Diagnosis and Treatment of Acute and Chronic Heart Failure 2008 of the European Society of Cardiology. Developed in collaboration with the Heart Failure Association of the ESC (HFA) and endorsed by the European Society of Intensive Care Medicine (ESICM) *European Journal of Heart Failure.* 2008;10(10):933–989.

[263] A Study Testing the Effectiveness of Nesiritide in Patients With Acute Decompensated Heart Failure, NCT00475852.

[264] Costanzo MR, Saltzberg MT, Jessup M, Teerlink JR, Sobotka PA. Ultrafiltration is associated with fewer rehospitalizations than continuous diuretic infusion in patients with decompensated heart failure: results from UNLOAD. *Journal of Cardiac Failure.* 2010;16(4):277–284.

[265] Arici M, Erdem Y. Dual blockade of the renin-angiotensin system for cardiorenal protection: an update. *American Journal of Kidney Diseases.* 2009;53(2):332–345.

[266] Arnold JMO, Howlett JG, Dorian P, et al. Canadian Cardiovascular Society Consensus Conference recommendations on heart failure update 2007. Prevention, management during intercurrent illness or acute decompensation, and use of biomarkers. *Canadian Journal of Cardiology.* 2007;23(1):21–45.

[267] Kazory A, Ross EA. Anemia: the point of convergence or divergence for kidney disease and heart failure? *Journal of the American College of Cardiology.* 2009;53(8):639–647.

[268] Sharma R, Francis DP, Pitt B, Poole-Wilson PA, Coats AJS, Anker SD. Haemoglobin predicts survival in patients with chronic heart failure: a substudy of the ELITE II trial. *European Heart Journal.* 2004;25(12):1021–1028.

In: Hemodialysis: Indications, Procedures and Complications ISBN: 978-1-62081-301-0
Editors: Y F. Cabral and M. Costa De Santos

Chapter II

Nutrition: From the Physiological Bases to Hemodialysis Patient Care

***Cláudia Rucco Penteado Detregiachi*[1], *Milene Peron Rodrigues Pinto*[2], *Maria Rita Marques de Oliveira*[3] *and Vânia Aparecida Leandro-Merhi*[4]**

[1]Universidade de Marília-SP, Unimar, Brazil
[2]Faculdade de Medicina da UNESP de Botucatu-SP, Brazil
[3]Instituto de Biociências da UNESP de Botucatu-SP, Brazil
[4]Pontificia Universidade Católica de Campinas-SP, Brazil

Abstract

Dialysis can worsen the nutritional status of dialysis patients and malnutrition worsens treatment prognosis. Hence, specific and personal nutritional therapy, with proper food intake, has a decisive role on the positive prognosis of chronic kidney disease patients undergoing hemodialysis. This chapter will cover the metabolic changes caused by chronic kidney disease which serve to guide appropriate nutritional therapy. The nutritional recommendations for the chronic kidney disease patient undergoing hemodialysis will be approached by their historical aspect and under the light of the current consensus and controversies. Assuming that appropriate food intake is challenging for the patient and for the healthcare team, the chapter will present a discussion on the etiological factors of inappropriate food intake by hemodialysis patients and the current strategies for overcoming this difficulty. Finally, the chapter will cover the perspectives and innovations of nutritional therapy during hemodialysis in order to improve food intake and the quality of life of hemodialysis patients.

1. Nutrient Metabolism in Chronic Renal Failure: Pathophysiological Bases for Nutritional Therapy

Nutritional and metabolic disorders are highly prevalent in chronic renal failure (CRF) patients regardless of treatment type, namely conservative treatment or dialysis (Bergstron et al., 1998), and significantly impact morbidity and mortality. However, interventions that improve the nutritional and metabolic status of CRF patients can improve their quality of life (Valderrábano et al., 2001, Castro et al., 2003), hence the importance of studies in this area.

Malnutrition in CRF is associated with many factors found in the pre-dialysis and dialysis phases, including influence of the underlying disease, inadequate food intake, psychosocial factors and altered macronutrient metabolism (Pupim et al., 2006).

In addition to its effect on water and electrolyte metabolism and on the acid-base balance, CRF induces a global change in energy metabolism and in the protein, fat, carbohydrate, mineral and vitamin metabolic pathways (Ikizler and Pupim, 2010).

Energy Metabolism

Total energy expenditure (TEE), which corresponds to the energy required by the body to carry out vital functions and physical activities, consists of the resting energy expenditure (REE), which is the energy spent while resting in bed under comfortable environmental conditions (60-75% of the TEE), food-induced thermogenesis, which is the thermal effect of foods (5-15% of the TEE) and energy spent on physical activities, which is considered the most variable component of TEE and can represent a significant amount of the energy spent by very active individuals (Institute of Medicine, 2002). In disease states, additional energy may be required to compensate high metabolic activity while low REE may result from cellular economization mechanisms caused by substrate unavailability. Additionally, the energy spent on physical activities may be low because of the compromised functional condition of the patient. Lean body mass, the most metabolically active component, is a first-line substrate for supplying additional energy during states of physiological stress. Although the amount of energy per unit of mass increases during stress, absolute REE decreases as body mass decreases. Hence, the estimated energy requirement of CRF patients depends on this equation of somewhat unpredictable variables. So, depending on the conditions of the study, REE can be positively (O'Sullivan et al., 2002, Panesar and Agarwal, 2003, Avesani et al., 2004) or negatively (Kuhlmann et al., 2001) associated with kidney function, or can even be similar to the REE of individuals without CRF (Schneeweiss et al., 1990, Kamimura et al., 2007a).

In CRF, REE corrected for unit of lean mass can be higher or lower than the REE of individuals without CRF. When CRF is stable, low REE per unit of lean mass can be explained by changes in cell metabolism characteristic of CRF (Om and Hohenegger, 1980, Conjard et al., 1995) and, especially, by the low cellular respiration of the kidneys, since the disease reduces blood flow to this organ (Kurnik et al., 1992). Note that approximately 25% of the cardiac output flows through the kidneys (Silva, 1987).

High REE in CRF patients is attributed to decompensated endocrine conditions (Mitch et al., 1999), inflammatory state, metabolic acidosis (Ikizler and Pupim, 2010), insulin resistance, secondary hyperparathyroidism and diabetes (Mitch et al., 1999). Inflammatory state is knowingly associated with high REE. In CRF patients who frequently experience an inflammatory state, high REE has been associated with high C-reactive protein and interleukin-6, two inflammatory markers (Kamimura et al. 2007a, 2007b). Sepsis has also been associated with high REE (Schneeweiss et al., 1990). Even dialysis has been associated with high REE (Pupim et al., 2006).

Clinically stable CRF patients under conservative treatment or dialysis usually have a REE similar to or slightly below that of healthy individuals matched by age and gender (Avesani et al., 2011). However, as mentioned above, when specific catabolic conditions are present, such as poorly controlled diabetes, hyperparathyroidism and inflammation, REE can be high.

Protein Metabolism

Metabolic acidosis is a frequent finding in CRF and stems from decreased glomerular filtration, which results in low excretion of hydrogen ions (Wiseman and Linas, 2005). Acidosis increases protein breakdown and reduces protein synthesis, resulting in muscle loss and negative nitrogen balance (Mehrotra et al., 2003, Kovacic et al., 2003, Szeto and Chow, 2004, Kraut and Kurtz, 2005, Du et al., 2005). Acidosis also seems to have an anti-anabolic action, but it is less intense than the stimulus for protein catabolism (Kalantar-Zadeh et al., 2004a). High protein catabolism is associated with insulin resistance and probably with high serum levels of cortisol (Bailey, 1998, Kopple et al., 2005, Du et al., 2005).

In metabolic acidosis, increased oxidation of branched-chain amino acids, such as isoleucine, leucine and valine, stimulates protein catabolism. This catabolic response results from increased branched-chain keto acid dehydrogenase (BCKD) activity evidenced by increased expression of the mRNA that codifies it (Kovacic et al., 2003, Szeto and Chow, 2004, Du et al., 2005). Another event responsible for muscle catabolism is the activation of the ubiquitin-proteasome proteolytic pathway. This is one of the main events that contribute for the breakdown of lean mass, actively increasing malnutrition in CRF patients with acidosis (Bailey, 1998, Franch and Mitch, 1998, Mitch, 2002, Du et al., 2005).

Hence, in CRF patients, hormonal changes and insulin resistance are responsible for low protein synthesis, while metabolic acidosis and inflammation are responsible for high protein catabolism, which result in malnutrition.

The treatment or prevention of acidosis can suppress muscle catabolism. This can be achieved by pharmaceutical drugs (Leite and Leal, 2002) or nutritional therapy (Chauveau et al., 2000, Remer, 2001).

Carbohydrate Metabolism

Insulin resistance (IR) is a frequently found complication in CRF patients, even in those on the first stages of the disease (Mak and DeFronzo, 1992), and is an important risk factor for cardiovascular diseases (Parfrey and Foley, 1999). IR manifests at the beginning of renal failure, even before uremic symptoms are evident, and improves significantly after dialysis (Kobayashi et al., 2000). This suggests that uremic toxins play an important role in IR.

Considering that insulin sensitivity correlates with the ability of the muscle to work in aerobic conditions, one may conclude that a sedentary lifestyle contributes to IR also in CRF patients, and this indicates that the insulin insensitivity of these patients improves with exercise (Goldberg et al., 1980).

The kidneys have a central role on insulin metabolism. This hormone is freely filtered, that is, the renal clearance of insulin is 200mL/minute, exceeding the glomerular filtration rate (GFR), which is 120mL/minute (Pupim et al., 2006). Thus, when GFR is low, insulin clearance is also low, causing hyperinsulinemia (Caravaca et al., 2010). The hyperparathyroidic state secondary to CRF is also implicated on the onset of IR since parathormone (PTH) inhibits the secretion of insulin by the pancreas (Chiu et al., 2000, Caravaca et al., 2010)

One of the functions of the active form of vitamin D, calcitriol, abbreviated as 1,25(OH)2D, is to stimulate the secretion of insulin by the pancreas (Bikle, 2010). Calcitriol deficiency is frequently present in CRF patients and may contribute to the low insulin secretion of these patients (Bikle, 2010).

Thus, because of insulin resistance, CRF patients can benefit from diets that encourage the consumption of complex carbohydrates since these facilitate the control of blood glucose and serum triglycerides. Both are usually high in CRF patients.

Lipid Metabolism

CRF patients have a high prevalence of cardiovascular diseases (CVD) which results in a mortality rate ten times higher than that of the general population (Tonelli et al., 2001). Studies show that this prevalence varies from 4.3 to 32% (Hiatt, 2001, Selvin and Erlinger, 2004, Leibson et al., 2004, Vinuesa et al., 2005).

Hyperlipidemia has been considered a risk factor for atherosclerotic disease in CRF patients. It is characterized by hypercholesterolemia, low HDL and especially, hypertriglyceridemia (Green et al., 1983, Gomez Dumm et al., 2001; Aragão et al., 2009). Dialysis seems to act as an adjuvant for the development of hypertriglyceridemia. The serum triglyceride levels of CRF patients undergoing dialysis are 50% higher than those of patients receiving conservative treatment (Hahn et al., 1983). The delayed catabolism of lipoproteins high in triglycerides is the metabolic change that promotes the genesis of dyslipidemia in CRF, resulting in high serum levels of very low-density lipoprotein cholesterol (VLDL-C) and low-density lipoprotein cholesterol (LDL-C) and low serum levels of high-density lipoprotein cholesterol (HDL-C) (Samuelsson et al., 1991). Dyslipidemia in CRF patients is frequently associated with accumulation of visceral fat and the metabolic syndrome (Eckel et al., 2005).

Other risk factors are also associated with CVD in CRF patients, such as high blood pressure, diabetes mellitus and smoking (Aragão et al., 2009). Less common factors which seem to have a relevant role in the development of the atherosclerotic process in these patients have recently been described, such as inflammation, oxidative stress, persistent infection, proteinuria and hyperphosphatemia (Shlipak et al., 2005).

CRF patients have high serum concentrations of inflammatory markers, such as C-reactive protein (CRP) and interleukin 6 (IL-6) (Stenvinkel, 2006). Evidence suggests that chronic inflammation is critical for the development and progression of atherosclerosis in

CRF patients (Ross, 1999, Kaysen, 2001, Papagianni et al., 2003). Dietary interventions that modulate serum lipoprotein profiles, vascular endothelial function and the inflammatory response can help in the metabolic control of CRF patients.

Mineral and Vitamin Metabolism

The kidneys play a crucial role in the maintenance of the water and electrolyte balance. In CRF, changes in water and electrolyte homeostases impact the morbidity of CRF patients significantly.

The serum concentration of certain minerals can change because of the reduced GFR, anorexia, use of restrictive diets, contamination from the water used in dialysis, malabsorption, increased body excretions and losses, and the use of pharmaceutical drugs that affect mineral metabolism (Zima et al., 1996).

The ability to excrete sodium and potassium is hindered when GFR decreases significantly (<15 mL/minute) (Ikizler and Pupim, 2010).

Disorders in calcium and phosphorus metabolism involve mainly the hormones PTH and calcitriol and can lead to renal osteodystrophy (Drueke, 1998). CRF causes hyperphosphatemia, calcitriol deficiency and secondary hyperparathyroidism (Ikizler and Pupim, 2010). Changes in calcium metabolism found in CRF patients is caused by many factors, one of them being uremia, which reduces albumin's affinity for calcium (Suki and Rouse, 1991), and another being low intestinal absorption of calcium due to calcitriol deficiency (Ikizler and Pupim, 2010). The factors that contribute to hyperparathyroidism in CRF patients are low calcium concentration, phosphate retention, changes in vitamin D activation, uremic toxicity and low PTH catabolism (Suki and Rouse, 1991). High serum levels of phosphorus stem mainly from three factors: excessive intake of this mineral, especially by those consuming too much protein, low phosphorus excretion because of low GFR and bone remodeling (Alvestrand, 1990). As GFR decreases, the kidneys adapt and this adaptation is characterized by reduced tubular reabsorption of phosphorus, thereby increasing phosphaturia. However, when GFR < 25mL/minute, high PTH levels inhibit phosphaturia, causing hyperphosphatemia (Slatopolsky and Bricker, 1993).

The kidneys play an important role in the activation of vitamin D. For vitamin D to become active, it requires a last hydroxylation that occurs in the proximal convoluted tubules of the kidneys by action of the enzyme 1-α hydroxylase. The end product is 1,25 dihydroxyvitamin D3, [1,25(OH)2D] or calcitriol (Audran, 1985). In CRF, low phosphate excretion by the kidneys reduces the activity of 1-α hydroxylase and consequently, calcitriol deficiency (Kumar, 2011). However, low serum calcium levels stimulate the synthesis of calcitriol by increasing PTH secretion. Another important mechanism in the regulation of 1-α hydroxylase is the serum level of calcitriol, whose synthesis is controlled by feedback (Kumar, 2011). Although vitamin D deficiency is not a common finding in CRF patients, the use of this vitamin is indicated for the treatment of secondary hyperparathyroidism present in the final stage of CRF (Hansen et al., 2009).

Anemia is found in most CRF patients and is caused mainly by low production of erythropoietin due to uremic toxins, which also reduce erythrocyte half-life (Mafra and Cozzolino, 2000). Folic acid or vitamin B12 deficiency and restriction of high-protein foods, which are also sources of dietary iron, are among the causes of anemia in CRF (Ikizler and Pupim, 2010).

Zinc deficiency in CRF is also reported in the literature, especially in patients submitted to hemodialysis (Mafra and Cozzolino, 2000). Iron-deficiency anemia can increase the concentration of zinc protoporphyrin and thereby change the concentrations of zinc in the plasma and erythrocytes (Mafra and Cozzolino, 2000).

2. Nutritional Recommendations for Chronic Renal Failure Patients Undergoing Hemodialysis

Nutritional therapy (NT) is extremely important for the maintenance of adequate nutrient intake and helps to prevent and treat common comorbidities, such as water retention, high blood pressure, hyperkalemia and hyperphosphatemia (Kalantar-Zadek et al., 2004b, Kamimura et al., 2007a). The objectives of NT in these patients are: to recover and/or maintain adequate nutritional status, minimize protein catabolism, maintain the acid-base balance, maintain adequate levels of water, electrolytes, minerals and vitamins and improve the prognosis (Martins et al., 2011, Araujo et al., 2006).

Recommendations for Energy

Studies on metabolic balance have shown that stable CRF patients undergoing dialysis who are mildly physically active and consume an appropriate amount of proteins daily have a neutral nitrogen balance when their energy intake is about 35kcal/kg/day. For patients older than 60 years, 30kcal/kg/day seem to be enough (Fouque et al., 2007). Obese patients or patients with visceral obesity or the metabolic syndrome may need a lower energy intake to reduce fat mass and improve glucose tolerance and lipid abnormalities (Kumagai, 2007).

Recommendations for Proteins

CRF patients undergoing hemodialysis have a higher protein requirement than healthy individuals (Fouque et al., 2007), since dialysis causes protein loss and catabolism (Ikizler et al., 1994, Combarnous et al., 2002, Lim et al., 2005).

According to studies that directly assessed the protein requirement of patients undergoing hemodialysis and many guidelines, such as the Nutritional Guidelines of the National Kidney Foundation – Kidney Disease Outcomes Quality Initiative (NKF-KDOQI)(2002), roughly 1.2 grams of protein/kilo of body weight/day are necessary for obtaining a neutral or positive nitrogen balance in most clinically stable CRF patients. The protein requirement of malnourished patients is slightly higher, ranging from 1.2 to 1.4 grams/kg/day. In both cases, at least 50% of the proteins consumed should be of high biological value.

Recommendations for Carbohydrates and Fats

The recommended percentage of dietary energy coming from carbohydrates and fats for these patients is the same as that for healthy individuals, that is, 50 to 60% of the energy should come from carbohydrates and about 25% should come from fats. Complex carbohydrates should be preferred because their high dietary fiber content improves insulin action and glucose homeostasis. The preferred fats are those that contribute to an appropriate serum lipoprotein profile. Dietary fats should consist mostly of mono- and polyunsaturated fats, including omega-3 fatty acids, keeping saturated fats to a minimum (Kalantar-Zadeh et al., 2003).

Recommendations for Fluids and Minerals

Fluids: Urine volume is an excellent guide for establishing ideal fluid intake. An increase of 2 to 4.5% of the dry weight is safe for most patients (NKF-KDOQI, 2002). The recommended fluid intake is 500mL + the urinary volume produced in 24 hours (Wiggins et al., 2002).

Sodium: Sodium intake by hemodialysis patients increase their thirst and promotes water retention, resulting in interdialytic weight gain, which is always of great concern for the clinical hemodialysis team since an excessive weight gain may expose the patient to high risk of heart failure and the quick removal of the excess water during hemodialysis may induce severe hypotension, angina and cramps (Tomson, 2001). In most patients, a sodium intake of 2 to 3 grams/day results in good clinical outcome (Wiggins et al., 2002, Beto and Bansal, 2004). Patients with low energy intake and no clinical manifestations of excess water retention do not have to restrict sodium intake so severely, especially during the last meal before dialysis, which is usually 7 to 9 hours before the procedure (Martins et al., 2011).

Potassium: Patients with a urine volume of 1,000mL/day or more usually do not need to restrict potassium intake. Serum levels of potassium should be measured regularly to restrict intake, if necessary (Martins et al., 2011). In general, hemodialysis patients should consume 40mg of potassium per kilo of body weight per day (Wiggins et al., 2002). One way to reduce the amount of potassium in vegetables and fruits is to chop them in small pieces, soak them in water for some time, discard the water and boil them a few times, always changing the water (Copetti et al., 2010).

Phosphorus: High serum phosphorus is common in hemodialysis patients. When this happens, dietary phosphorus should be restricted to ideally less than 800mg/day (Ahmad et al., 1997, Ikizler and Hakim, 1998, Wiggins et al., 2002). However, since these patients need to consume high levels of proteins, it is difficult to actually limit phosphorus intake, so the use of phosphate binders may be necessary (Martins et al., 2011).

Calcium: Calcium intake by dialysis patients should range from 1,000 to 1,500 mg/day (Ahmad et al., 1997, Ikizler and Hakim, 1998, Wiggins et al., 2002). Calcium supplementation may be necessary because of low intestinal absorption and frequent restriction of dairy products because of their high phosphorus content.

Recommendations for Vitamins

Vitamin deficiencies in CRF patients are common and secondary to inadequate food intake, restrictive diets and depletion caused by pharmaceutical drugs (Steiber and Kopple, 2011). There are only a few studies on the vitamin requirements of CRF patients, and the recommended amounts are usually the same as those for healthy individuals.

Fat-soluble vitamins: Except for vitamin D, supplementation of fat-soluble vitamins is not recommended, especially of vitamin A, since it may accumulate in the body (NKF-KDOQI, 2002). The active form of vitamin D (1,25-hydrocholecalciferol) can be recommended to increase intestinal absorption of calcium, prevent and treat hyperparathyroidism and improve bone metabolism. Supplementation will depend on serum levels of calcium, phosphorus and PTH (Hultberg et al., 1993, Ahmad et al., 1997, Ikizler and Hakim, 1998). Vitamin E supplementation in CRF patients at risk of cardiovascular events is contraindicated (Kalantar-Zadeh and Kopple, 2003, Steiber and Kopple, 2011).

Water-soluble vitamins: The Dialysis Outcome Practice Patterns Study showed that the mortality of dialysis patients supplementing with water-soluble vitamins is 16% lower than that of patients who do not supplement on these vitamins. This fact holds even after adjustment for age, gender, race, comorbidities, hemoglobin, albumin, BMI and other possibly confounding factors (Fisell et al., 2004).

In addition to the usually low dietary intake of water-soluble vitamins, these vitamins are also lost during dialysis. Supplementation is recommended, especially of the vitamin B complex (folic acid and pyridoxine) and vitamin C. Homocysteine is a potent atherosclerotic agent and its serum levels are usually high in CRF patients (Hultberg et al., 1993), which happens to be correlated with early vascular disease. Vitamins B12, B6 and folic acid function as co-factors in the enzymatic reactions of homocysteine metabolism. Pharmacological doses of these vitamins taken daily reduce the serum homocysteine levels of CRF patients (Arnadottir et al., 1993, Kalantar-Zadeh and Kopple, 2003).

In CRF, supplementation of vitamin B6 is necessary, especially by individuals with inadequate food intake or those using certain pharmaceutical drugs. The European Society of Parenteral and Enteral Nutrition, and Caring for Australians with Renal Insufficiency Guidelines advise dialysis patients to take 5 mg/day of vitamin B6. Kalantar-Zadeh and Kopple (2003) reported that CRF patients undergoing hemodialysis respond well and quickly to vitamin B12 supplementation, even if their serum B12 levels are normal.

3. Food Intake of Hemodialysis Patients: Challenges and Strategies

Malnutrition is highly prevalent in CRF patients, both during the pre-dialysis (Lawson et al., 2001) and dialysis phases (Cuppari et al., 1989, Bergstrom and Lindhom, 1993), and is an important predictor of morbidity and mortality in this population.

In CRF, malnutrition may stem from inadequate food intake or have as predominant etiological factors the metabolic changes, inflammation and comorbidities secondary to the disease (Stenvinkel et al., 2000).

High levels of inflammatory markers, such as acute phase proteins and proinflammatory cytokines, have a marked influence on nutritional status since they induce anorexia and weight loss, which is secondary to protein catabolism and low anabolism (Kaizu et al., 1998, Bergstrom, 1999). In CRF, the levels of these markers are high and inversely correlated with renal function (Axelsson et al., 2006, Kamimura et al., 2007b). Interleukin-6 and TNF-α act directly on protein metabolism and indirectly on the central nervous system, causing anorexia.

According to Stenvinkel (2005), inflammation and metabolic acidosis may hinder protein anabolism, regardless of food intake.

Hypoalbuminemia is a common finding in CRF and is associated with higher risk of mortality in this population (Fouque et al., 2008). It is possible but not proven that the deficiency of this protein may predispose the patient to inflammatory states (Ling et al., 2004).

In addition to anorexia and inflammation, other conditions are cited in the literature as promoters of lean mass loss in CRF patients. These conditions include intercurrent catabolic diseases (Grodstein et al., 1980); loss of nutrients in the dialysate (Chazot et al., 1997); uremia (Kalantar-Zadeh et al., 2004b); endocrine disorders, such as insulin resistance (Mak, 1996) and growth hormone (Moyle et al., 2004); hyperparathyroidism (Kopple et al., 1980) and loss of blood (Kaplan et al., 1995).

Anorexia is relatively common in CRF patients undergoing hemodialysis (Bossola et al., 2005, Bossola et al., 2006). Some mechanisms have been suggested for explaining anorexia in CRF patients, such as changes in the levels of the hormones leptin and ghrelin and in neuropeptide Y (NPY) (Carrero et al., 2008). Leptin is released by adipose tissue and one of its actions is to reduce hunger by inhibiting NPY. CRF patients have high levels of leptin, which may result in anorexia (Mak et al., 2006). Ghrelin, an orexigenic peptide released by gastric cells, regulates body weight by controlling the centers of hunger and energy balance (Wynne et al., 2005). Higher levels of ghrelin in hemodialysis patients than controls are a common finding (Chan et al., 2005), possibly also promoting anorexia in uremic patients.

Figure 1 shows the set of factors that impact the nutritional status of CRF patients undergoing dialysis. Low nutrient intake is the main factor, but not the only factor. There are metabolic and treatment-related factors that may deplete the body's nutrient reserves.

Dyspeptic complaints are also common in CRF patients, such as nausea, vomiting, feeling of stomach fullness and epigastric pain (Van Vlen et al., 2001, Hirako et al., 2005). These complaints may be associated with delayed gastric emptying, which is caused by neuropathy (Dimitrascu et al., 1995), metabolic acidosis or anemia (Hirako et al., 2005), also common in CRF.

CRF patients emerge as the main elements of this very complex scenario involving physiological and emotional factors that are difficult to control. What are the necessary strategies for providing effective nutritional care? The first step involves the social, cultural and cognitive contextualization of the CRF patient, followed by appropriate assessment of his/her nutritional status and food intake. Helping patients to understand the extent and the reasons for their low food intake is extremely important for getting them to participate actively in the planning of their nutritional care scheme, making them capable of exposing their opinions on the decisions that regard proper food intake. Effective and empathetic communication with CRF patients and monitoring of their anthropometric measurements, food intake, biochemical markers of nutritional and metabolic statuses, and quality of life will act as indicators of results, and may confirm or redirect care-related strategies.

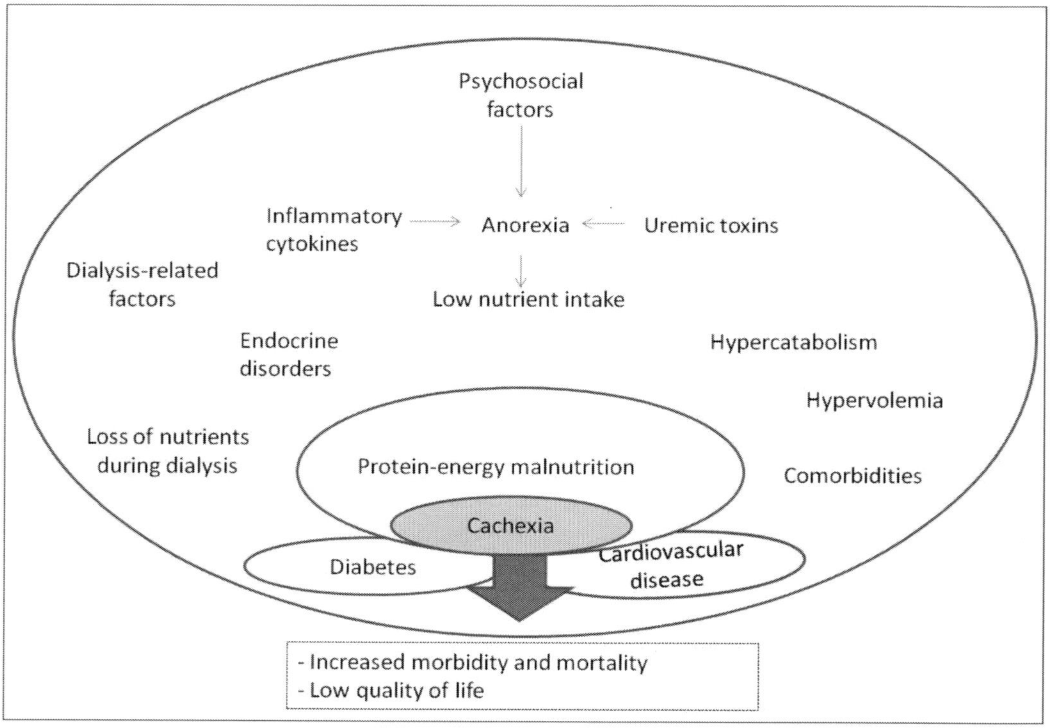

Figure 1. Representation of the causes of malnutrition in CRF.

4. Perspectives and Innovations Regarding Nutritional Therapy for Hemodialysis Patients

In addition to focusing care on the person and taking into account his or her context of life with CRF, his or her support network, wealth, psychological conditions, among others variables of global order, care of CRF patients can be complemented with therapeutic innovations, some whose outcomes are still being confirmed by scientific studies.

Growth hormone (GH) has been indicated to circumvent the loss of lean mass or even cachexia, which will help to reduce morbidity and mortality associated with low protein reserves (Van Der Sluis et al., 2000, Hansen et al., 2000, Haffner et al., 2000, Hokken-Koelega et al., 2000, Feldt-Rasmussen et al., 2007). Considering that GH promotes anabolism (Eisemann et al., 1989; Haymond and Mauras, 1996, Kopple et al., 2005), even in uremic patients (Kova´cs et al., 1996, Kopple et al., 2005), whether pediatric (Haffner et al., 2000, Hokken-Koelega et al., 2000) or adult (Hansen et al., 2000, Feldt-Rasmussen et al., 2007), the use of this hormone would benefit patients with CRF. GH increases muscle mass and bone mineral density, reduces fat mass and induces corresponding biochemical changes (Van Der Sluis et al., 2000)

A study called OPPORTUNITY™ (Kopple et al., 2011) followed 695 CRF patients undergoing hemodialysis for 20 weeks and found that, compared with patients taking placebo, patients taking GH lost weight and body fat and experienced a decrease in serum C-reactive protein and homocysteine levels and an increase in serum HDL-C and transferrin levels.

However, given the magnitude of the differences, these findings need to be confirmed by additional studies.

Another indication for using GH is delayed growth secondary to CRF. Studies with CRF patients taking GH, regardless of treatment type, that is, dialysis, conservative treatment or transplanted kidney, concluded that this is a safe therapeutic option with beneficial effects (Ulinski and Cochat, 2006, Vimalanchandra et al., 2006, Williams, 2006, Mahesh and Kaskel, 2008, Gorman and Frankenfield, 2008). However, the National Kidney Foundation (NKF) (2002) recommends correcting nutritional deficiencies and metabolic changes before considering treatment with GH.

Carnitine (3-hydroxy-4-N,N,N-trimethylaminobutyrate) is a quaternary amine synthesized by the liver, kidneys and brain from the essential amino acids lysine and methionine. Its synthesis requires iron, ascorbic acid, niacin and vitamin B6 (Evans and Fornasi, 2003). Carnitine is required for the transport of free fatty acids from the cytosol to the mitochondria, facilitating their oxidation and generating adenosine triphosphate in the energy metabolic pathway (Mitchell, 1978). Dialysis may cause loss of carnitine (Ahamad, 2001). Furthermore, carnitine deficiency in CRF patients may stem from low carnitine intake or low intake of its precursor amino acids (lysine and methionine), intestinal malabsorption, reduced synthesis in the kidneys, abnormal transport, low activity of the enzymes involved in the carnitine system and increased requirement (Ahamad, 2001, Guarnieri et al., 2001, Locatelli et al., 2002). Low carnitine levels in the body may cause cell disorders, including impaired fatty acid oxidation and energy production, deterioration of the lipid profile, accumulation of toxic products of fat metabolism and inhibition of some enzymes of the metabolic pathway (Brass et al., 2001). Some authors suggest that hemodialysis patients should take carnitine supplements (Golper et al., 2003, Sotirakopoulos et al., 2000, Vesel´a et al., 2001). Others suggest that this supplementation should only be recommended when dialysis patients do not respond to conventional therapies (Reuter et al., 2007) since the outcomes of carnitine supplementation vary widely. The recommended carnitine dosage for hemodialysis patients ranges from 5 to 100mg/kg, administered intravenously, orally or through dialysis (Kletzmayr et al., 1999, Ahamad, 2001).

Strategies that include frequent dialysis sessions, nutritional counseling and pharmaceutical-drug therapy have been proposed to circumvent anorexia in CRF patients (Bossola et al., 2009). Megestrol acetate, a synthetic substance obtained from progesterone, can enhance appetite by stimulating the production of NPY and inhibiting the production of pro-inflammatory cytokines, such as interleukin-1, interleukin-6 and TNF-α (Bossola et al., 2005). Studies with hemodialysis patients found that this substance increases their appetite, promotes weight gain and increases serum albumin levels. The recommended dosages vary from 40 to 800 mg/day (Lien and Ruffenach, 1996, Boccanfuso et al., 2000, Costero et al., 2004, Rammohan et al., 2005). However, these results do not yet serve as ground for clinical practice since they do not stem from controlled and randomized trials (Bossola et al., 2009).

A studied strategy to minimize anorexia in CRF patients is supplementation with branched-chain amino acids (BCAA) (AACR) (Hiroshige et al., 2001). These authors used a randomized, placebo-controlled study to verify the effects of a 12g/day supplementation of BCAA in 28 malnourished patients with hypoalbuminemia and found that they improved significantly compared with controls because their serum levels of these amino acids returned to normal. Another promising perspective in the context of anorexia is the administration of ghrelin to induce weight gain and reduce pro-inflammatory cytokine levels (Anderstam et al., 1996, Schmid et al., 2005, Druce et al., 2006).

Oxidative stress is common in hemodialysis patients (Massy and Nguyen-Khoa, 2002) and is associated with a significant reduction in their antioxidant capacity. Hence, antioxidant therapies have been proposed in the literature. Studies with hemodialysis patients have investigated supplementation with roughly 800 IU/day of vitamin E (α-tocopherol) (Islam et al., 2000, Roob et al., 2000, Lu et al., 2007) but these authors state that more studies are needed before this procedure is incorporated by clinical practice.

Vitamin C is another substance with antioxidant activity that has been recommended for hemodialysis patients. The recommended weekly dosage is 1 to 1.5 grams of ascorbic acid orally or 300mg parenterally in each hemodialysis session (Deicher and Horl, 2003, Fumeron et al., 2005), but this initiative also requires further studies.

Final Considerations

CRF patients, especially those undergoing hemodialysis, have a complex pathophysiology. The dietary restrictions usually necessary for hemodynamic balance may cause malnutrition. Diets for CRF patients should contain proper amounts of energy and nutrients, with special attention to electrolyte homeostasis. Consumption of proteins and water-soluble vitamins should also be above average. However, as the patient's health deteriorates, anorexia secondary to multiple causes is the main factor limiting adequate food intake. A holistic treatment that focuses on the person is the main strategy for facing the problem, but one should not disregard all the therapeutic innovations.

References

Ahmad, KR.; Kopple, JD. Chapter - Nutrition in maintenance hemodialysis patients. In: Kopple, JD; Massry, SG; eds. *Nutritional management of renal disease.* New York: Williams and Wilkins; 1997; p. 563-93.

Ahamad, S. L-Carnitine in Dialysis Patients. *Semin. Dial.*, 2001; 14(3), 209-17.

Alvestrand, A. Protein metabolism and nutrition in hemodialysis patients control. *Nefrology*, 1990; 78, 102-18.

Anderstam, B; Mamoun, A; Sodersten, P; et al. Middle-sizes molecule fractions isolated from uremic ultrafiltrate and normal urine inhibit ingestive behaviour in the rat. *J. Am. Soc. Nephrol.*, 1996; 7, 2453-2460.

Aragão, JA; Reis, FP; Borges Neto, RR; Aragão, MECS; Nunes, MAP; Feitosa, VLC. Prevalência da doença arterial obstrutiva periférica em doentes com insuficiência renal crônica. *J. Vasc. Bras.*, 2009; 8(4), 301-306.

Araujo, IC; Kamimura, MA; Draibe, AS; et al. Nutritional parameters and mortality in incident hemodialysis patients. *J. Ren. Nutr.*, 2006; 16, 27-35.

Arnadottir, M; Brattstrom, L; Simonsen, O; et al. The effect of high-dose pyridoxine and folic acid supplementation on serum lipid and plasma homocysteine concentrations in dialysis patients. *Clin. Nephrol.*, 1993; 40, 236-40.

Audran, M. The physiology and pathophysiology of vitamin D. *Mayo Clin. Proc.*, 1985; 60, 851-866.

Avesani, CM; Draibe, SA; Kamimura, MA; Colugnati, FA; Cuppari, L. Resting energy expenditure of chronic kidney disease patients: influence of renal function and subclinical inflammation. *Am. J. Kidney Dis.*, 2004; 44(6), 1008-16.

Avesani, CM; Kamimura, MA; Cuppari, L. Energy expenditure in chronic kidney disease patients. *J. Ren. Nutr.*, 2011; 21(1), 27-30.

Axelsson, J; Heimburger, O; Stenvinkel, P. Adipose tissue and inflammation in chronic kidney disease. *Contrib. Nephrol.*, 2006; 151, 165-74.

Bailey, JL. Metabolic acidosis and protein catabolism: mechanisms and clinical implications. *Miner. Electrolyte Metab.*, 1998; 24(1), 13-9.

Bergstron, J; Wang, T; Lindholm, B. Factors contributing to catabolism in end-stage renal disease patients. *Miner. Electrolyte Metab.*, 1998; 24, 92-101.

Bergstrom, J. Mechanisms of uremic suppression of appetite. *J. Ren. Nutr.*, 1999; 9(3), 129-32.

Bergstrom, J; Lindhom, B. Nutrition and adequacy of dialysis. How do hemodialysis and CAPD compare? *Kidney Int.*, 1993; 43, 439-550.

Beto, JA; Bansal, VK. Medical nutrition therapy in chronic kidney failure: integrating clinical practice guidelines. *J. Am. Diet Assoc.*, 2004; 104, 404–409.

Bikle, DD. Vitamin D: newly discovered actions require reconsideration of physiologic requirements. *Trends Endocrinol. Metab.*, 2010; 21(6), 375-384.

Boccanfuso, JA; Hutton, M; McAllister, B. The effects of megestrol acetate on nutritional parameters in a dialysis population. *J. Ren. Nutr.*, 2000; 10,36-43.

Bossola, M; Tazza, L; Luciani, G. Mechanisms and Treatment of Anorexia in End-Stage Renal Disease Patients on Hemodialysis. *Journal of Renal Nutrition*, 2009; 19(1), 2–9.

Bossola, M; Muscaritoli, M; Tazza, L; et al. Malnutrition in hemodialysis patients: what therapy? *Am. J. Kidney Dis*, 2005; 46, 371-386.

Bossola, M; Tazza, L. Giungi, S; et al. Anorexia in hemodialysis patients: an update. *Kidney Int*, 2006; 70, 417-422.

Brass, EP; Adler, S; Sietsema, KE; Hiatt, WR; Orlando, AM; Amato, A. Intravenous L-carnitine increases plasma carnitine, reduces fatigue and may preserve exercise capacity in hemodialysis patients. *Am. J. Kidney Dis.*, 2001; 37(5), 1018-28.

Caravaca, F; Cerezo, I; Macías, R; García de Vinuesa, E; Martínez del Viejo, C; Villa, J; Martínez Gallardo, R; Ferreira, F; Hernández-Gallego, R. Insulin resistance in chronic kidney disease: its clinical characteristics and prognostic significance. *Nefrologia*, 2010; 30(6), 661-8.

Carrero, JJ; Aguilera, A; Stenvinkel, P; et al. Appetite disorders in uremia. *J. Ren. Nutr*, 2008; 18, 107-113.

Castro, M; Caiuby, AVS; Draibe, SA; Canziani, MEF. Qualidade de vida de pacientes com insuficiência renal crônica em hemodiálise avaliada através do instrumento genérico SF-36. *Rev. Assoc. Med. Bras.*, 2003; 49(3), 245-9.

Chan, CC; Hung, CH; Yen, CS; et al. The relationship of plasma ghrelin level to energy regulation, feeling and left ventricular function in non-diabetic hemodialysis patients. *Nephrol. Dial Transplant*, 2005; 20, 2172-2177.

Chauveau, P; Fouque, D; Combe, C; Laville, M; Canaud, B; Azar, R; et al. Acidosis and status nutritional in hemodialyzed patients. French Study Group for Nutrition in Dialysis. *Semin. Dial.*, 2000; 13(4), 241-6.

Chazot, C; Shahmir, E; Matias, B; et al. Dialytic nutrition: provision of amino acids in dialysate during hemodialysis. *Kidney Int.*, 1997; 52, 1663–1670.

Chiu, KC; Chuang, LM; Lee, NP; Ryu, JM; McGullam, JL; Tsai, GP; Saad, MF. Insulin sensitivity is inversely correlated with plasma intact parathyroid hormone level. *Metabolism.*, 2000; 49(11), 1501-5.

Combarnous, F; Tetta, C; Cellier, CC; et al. Albumin loss in on-line hemodiafiltration. *Int. J. Artif. Organs.*, 2002; 25, 203–209.

Conjard, A; Ferrier, B; Martin, M; Caillette, A; Carrier, H; Baverel, G. Effects of chronic renal failure on enzymes of energy metabolism in individual human muscle fibers. *J. Am. Soc. Nephrol.*, 1995; 6(1), 68-74.

Copetti, C; Oliveira, VR; Kirinus, P. Avaliação da redução de potássio em hortaliças submetidas a diferentes métodos de cocção para possível utilização na dietoterapia renal. *Revista Nutrição de Campinas*, 2010; 23(5), 831-838.

Costero, O; Bajo, MA; Del Peso, G; et al. Treatment of anorexia and malnutrition in peritoneal dialysis patients with megestrol acetate. *Adv. Periton. Dial*, 2004; 20, 209-212.

Cuppari, L; Draibe, SA; Ançäo, MS; Sigulem, D; Sustovich, DR; Ajzen, H; Ramos, OL. Avaliação nutricional em pacientes renais crônicos em programa de hemodiálise: estudo multicêntrico. *AMB.*, 1989; 35(1), 9-14.

Deicher, R; Horl, WH. Vitamin C in chronic kidney disease and hemodialysis patients. *Kidney Blood Press Res*, 2003; 26, 100–106.

Dimitrascu, DL; Barnet, J; Kirschner, T; Wienbeck, M. Astral emptying of semisolid meal measured by real-time ultrasonography in chronic renal failure. *Dig. Dis. Sci.*, 1995; 40, 636-44.

Druce, MR; Neary, NM; Small, CJ; et al. Subcutaneous administration of ghrelin stimulates energy intake in healthy lean human volunteers. *Int. J. Obes*, 2006; 30, 293-296.

Drueke, T.B. Anomalies of phosphate and calcium metabolism in cgronic renal insufficiency. *Rev. Prat.*, 1998; 48, 1207-12.

Du, Z; Hu, D; Mitch, WE. Molecular mechanisms activating muscle protein degradation in chronic kidney disease and other catabolic conditions. *Eur. J. Clin. Invest.*, 2005; 35(3), 157-63.

Eckel, RH; Grundy, SM; Zimmet, PZ. The metabolic syndrome. *Lancet*, 2005; 365(9468), 1415-28.

Eisemann, JH; Hammond, AC; Rumsey, TS. Tissue protein synthesis and nucleic acid concentrations in steers treated with somatotropin. *Br. J. Nutr*, 1989; 62, 657–671.

Evans, AG; Fornasi, G. Pharmacokinetics of L-Carnitine. *Clin. Pharmacokinet.*, 2003; 42(11), 941-67.

Feldt-Rasmussen, B; Lange, M; Sulowicz, W; et al. Growth hormone treatment during hemodialysis in a randomized trial improves nutrition, quality of life, and cardiovascular risk. *J. Am. Soc. Nephrol*, 2007; 18, 2161–2171.

Fissell, RB; Bragg-Gresham, JL; Gillespie, BW; et al. International variation in vitamin prescription and association with mortality in the Dialysis Outcomes and Practice Patterns Study (DOPPS). *Am. J. Kidney Dis.*, 2004; 44(2), 293-9.

Fouque, D; Vennegoor, M; Wee, PT; et al. EBPG Guideline on Nutrition. *Nephrol. Dial Transplant,* 2007; 22 (2), 45–87.

Fouque, D; Kalantar-Zadeh, K; Kopple, J; Cano, N; Chauveau, P; Cuppari, L; et al. A proposed nomenclature and diagnostic criteria for protein–energy wasting in acute and chronic kidney disease. *Kidney International*, 2008; 73, 391–398.

Franch, HA; Mitch, WE. Catabolism in uremia: the impact of metabolic acidosis. *J. Am. Soc. Nephrol.*, 1998; 9(suppl. 12), S78-S81.

Fumeron, C; Nguyen-Khoa, T; Saltiel, C; Kebede, M; Buisson, C; Dru¨ eke, TB; Lacour, B; Massy, ZA. Effects of oral vitamin C supplementation on oxidative stress and inflammation status in haemodialysis patients. *Nephrol. Dial Transplant*, 2005; 20, 1874–1879

Goldberg, AP; Hagberg, J; Delmez, JA; Carney, RM; et al. The catabolic and physiological effects of exercise training in hemosialysis patients. *Am. J. Clin. Nutr.*, 1980; 33, 1620-28.

Gomez Dumm, NT; Giammona, AM; Touceda, LA; Raimondi, C. Lipid abnormalities in chronic renal failure patients undergoing hemodialysis. *MEDICINA (Buenos Aires)* 2001; 61, 142-146.

Golper, TA; Goral, S; Becker, BN; et al. l-carnitine treatment of anemia. *Am. J. Kidney Dis.*, 2003; 41(Suppl 4), S27–S34.

Gorman, G; Frankenfield, D. Linear growth in pediatric hemodialysis patients. *Pediatr. Nephrol.*, 2008; 23, 123-7.

Green, D; Stone, NJ; Krumlowsky, A. Putative atherogenic factors in patients with chronic renal failure. *Prog. Cardiovasc. Dis*, 1983; 26, 133-44.

Grodstein, GP; Blumenkrantz, MJ; Kopple, JD. Nutritional and metabolic response to catabolic stress in uremia. *Am. J. Clin. Nutr*, 1980; 33, 1411–1416.

Guarnieri, G; Situlin, R; Biolo, G. Carnitine metabolism in uremia. *Am. J. Kidney Dis.*, 2001; 38(4 Suppl 1), S63-7.

Hahn, R; Oette, K; Mondorf, H; Finke, K; Sieberth, HG. Analysis of cardiovascular risk factors in chronic hemodialysis patients with special attention to the hyperlipoproteinemias. *Atherosclerosis*, 1983; 48, 279-88.

Haffner, D; Schaefer, F; Nissel, R; et al. Effect of growth hormone treatment on the adult height of children with chronic renal failure. German Study Group for Growth Hormone Treatment in Chronic Renal Failure. *N. Engl. J. Med*, 2000; 343, 923–930.

Hansen, D; Brandi, L; Rasmussen, K. Treatment of secondary hyperparathyroidism in haemodialysis patients: a randomised clinical trial comparing paricalcitol and alfacalcidol. *BMC Nephrol.*, 2009; 24, 10:28.

Hansen, TB; Gram, J; Jensen, PB; et al. Influence of growth hormone on whole body and regional soft tissue composition in adult patients on hemodialysis. A double-blind, randomized, placebo-controlled study. *Clin. Nephrol*, 2000; 53, 99–107.

Haymond, MW; Mauras, N. The rationale for the use of recombinant human growth hormone and insulin-like growth factor-I for catabolic conditions in humans. *Horm. Res,* 1996; 46, 202–207.

Hiatt, WR. Medical treatment of peripheral arterial disease and claudication. *N. Engl. J. Med.*, 2001; 344, 1608-21.

Hirako, M; Misu, N; Kobayashi, Y; Adachi, H; Shikano, M; Matsuhisa, E; Kimura, G. Impaired gastric motility and its relationship to gastrointestinal syntoms in patients with chronic renal failure. *J. Gastroenterol.*, 2005; 40(12), 1116-22.

Hiroshige, K; Sonta, T; Suda, T; et al. Oral supplementation of branched chain amino acid improves nutritional status in elderly patients on chronic hemodialysis. *Nephrol. Dial Transplant*, 2001; 16, 1856-1862.

Hokken-Koelega, A; Mulder, P; De Jong, R; et al. Long-term effects of growth hormone treatment on growth and puberty in patients with chronic renal insufficiency. *Pediatr. Nephrol.*, 2000; 14, 701–706.

Hultberg, B; Andersson, A; Sterner, G. Plasma homocysteine in renal failure. *Clin. Nephrol*, 1993; 40, 230-5.

Ikizler, A; Pupim, LB. Chapter 12 – Nutrition and Metabolism in Kidney Disease. In: Himmelfarb, Jonathan; Sayegh, Mohamed H. Chronic Kidney Disease, Dialysis, and Transplantation. 3rd ed. Elsevier Inc.; 2010; p.164-177.

Ikizler, TA; Flakoll, PJ; Parker, RA; et al. Amino acid and albumin losses during hemodialysis. *Kidney Int.*, 1994; 46, 830–837.

Ikizler, TA; Hakim, RM. Chapter - Nutritional requirements of hemodialysis patients. In: Mitch, WE; Klahr, S; eds. *Handbook of Nutrition and the Kidney*. Philadelphia: Lippincot-Raven; 1998; p. 253-68.

INSTITUTE OF MEDICINE (IOM). Dietary Reference Intakes for energy, carbohydrate, fiber, fat, fatty acids, cholesterol, *protein, and amino acids (Macronutrients).* Washington, D.C.: National Academy Press; 2002.

Islam, KN; O'Byrne, D; Devaraj, S; Palmer, B; Grundy, SM; Jialal, I. Alpha-tocopherol supplementation decreases the oxidative susceptibility of LDL in renal failure patients on dialysis therapy. *Atherosclerosis*, 2000; 150, 217-224.

Kaizu, Y; Kimura, M; Yoneyama, T; Miyaji, K; Hibi, I; Kumagai, H. Interleukin-6 may mediate malnutrition in chronic hemodialysis patients. *Am. J. Kidney Dis.*, 1998; 31(1), 93-100.

Kalantar-Zadeh, K; Kopple, JD. Trace Elements and Vitamins in Maintenance Dialysis patients. *Advances in renal Replacement Therapy*, 2003; 10 (3), 170-182.

Kalantar-Zadeh, K; Block, G; Humphreys, MH; Kopple, JD. Reverse epidemiology of cardiovascular risk factors in maintenance dialysis patientes. *Kidney International*, 2003; 63, 793 – 808.

Kalantar-Zadeh, K; Mehrotra, R; Fouque, D; Kopple, JD. Metabolic acidosis and malnutrition inflammation complex syndrome in chronic renal failure. *Semin. Dial.*, 2004a; 17(6), 455-65.

Kalantar-Zadeh, K; Kopple, JD; Humphreys, MH; Block, G. Comparing outcome predictability of markers of malnutrition inflammation complex syndrome in haemodialysis patients. *Nephrol. Dial Transplant*, 2004b; 1507-19.

Kamimura, MA; Draibe, SA; Avesani, CM; Canziani, MEF; Colugnati, FAB; Cuppari, L. Resting energy expenditure and its determinants in hemodialysis patients. *Eur. J. Clin. Nutr.*, 2007a; 61(3), 362-7.

Kamimura, MA; Dalboni, MA; Draibe, SA; Avesani, CM; Cendoroglo, M; Canziani, MEF; et al. Serum and cellular interleukin-6 in hemodialysis patients: relationship with energy expenditure. *Nephrol. Dial Transpl.*, 2007b; 22, 839-44.

Kaplan, AA; Halley, SE; Lapkin, RA; et al. Dialysate protein losses with bleach processed polysulphone dialyzers. *Kidney Int.*, 1995; 47, 573–578.

Kaysen, GA. The microinflammatory state in uremia: causes and potential consequences. *J. Am. Soc. Nephrol.*, 2001; 12(7), 1549-57.

Kletzmayr, J; Mayer, G; Legenstein, E; et al. Anemia and carnitine supplementation in hemodialyzed patients. *Kidney Int.*, 1999; 55(Suppl 69), S93–S106.

Kobayashi, S; Maejima, S; Ikeda, T; Nogase, M. Impacto f dialysis therapy on insulin resistance in end-stage renal disease: comparison of haemodialysis and continous ambulatory peritoneal dialysis. *Nephrol. Dial. Transplant.*, 2000; 15(1), 65-70.

Kopple, JD; Cianciaruso, B; Massry, SG. Does parathyroid hormone cause protein wasting? *Contrib. Nephrol.*, 1980; 20, 138–148.

Kopple, JD; Kalantar-Zadeh, K; Mehrotra, R. Risks of chronic metabolic acidosis in patients with chronic kidney disease. *Kidney Int.*, 2005; 67(suppl 95), S21-S27.

Kopple, JD; Brunori, G; Leiserowitz, M; Fouque, D. Growth hormone induces anabolism in malnourished maintenance haemodialysis patients. *Nephrol. Dial Transplant*, 2005; 20, 952–958.

Kopple, JD; Cheung, AK; Christiansen, JS; et al. OPPORTUNITY: a large-scale randomized clinical trial of growth hormone in hemodialysis patients. *Nephrol. Dial Transplant*, 2011; 26, 4095–4103.

Kova´cs, GT; Oh, J; Kova´cs, J; et al. Growth promoting effects of growth hormone and IGF-I are additive in experimental uremia. *Kidney Int*, 1996; 49, 1413–1421.

Kovacic, V; Roguljic, L; Kovacic, V. Metabolic acidosis of chronically hemodialyzed patients. *Am. J. Nephrol.*, 2003; 23(3), 158-64.

Kraut, JA; Kurtz, I. Metabolic acidosis of CKD: diagnosis, clinical characteristics and treatment. *Am. J. Kidney Dis.*, 2005; 45(6), 978-93.

Kuhlmann, U; Schwickardi, M; Trebst, R; Lange, H. Resting metabolic rate in chronic renal failure. *J. Renal. Nutr.*, 2001; 11(4), 202-6.

Kumagai, H. Chapter - Nutritional Therapy for Patients Undergoing Hemodialysis. In: Suzuki, H; Kimmel, PL; eds. *Nutrition and Kidney Disease: A New Era. Contrib. Nephrol.* Basel, Karger; 2007; vol 155, p. 59-71.

Kumar, R. New clinical trials with vitamin D and analogs in renal disease. *Kidney International,* 2011; 80, 793-796.

Kurnik, BRC; Weisberg, LS; Kurnik, PB. Renal and systemic oxygen consumption in patients with normal and abnormal renal fucntion. *J. Am. Soc. Nephrol.*, 1992; 2(11), 1617-26.

Lawson, JA; Lazarus, R; Kelly, JJ. Prevalence and prognostic significance of malnutrition in chronic renal insufficiency. *J. Ren. Nutr.*, 2001; 11(1), 16-22.

Leibson, CL; Ransom, JE; Olson, W; Zimmerman, BR; O'fallon, WM; Palumbo, PJ. Peripheral arterial disease, diabetes, and mortality. *Diabetes Care*, 2004; 27, 2843-9.

Leite, MJr; Leal, E; Cardoso, LR. Correction of acidosis by hemodialysis: proposal of a correlation with urea kinetics. *Blood Purif.*, 2002; 20(6), 551-6.

Lien, YH; Ruffenach, SJ. Low dose megestrol increases serum albumin in malnourished dialysis patients. *Int. J. Artif. Organs*, 1996; 19, 147-150.

Lim, VS; Ikizler, TA; Raj, DS; et al. Does hemodialysis increase protein breakdown? Dissociation between whole-body amino acid turnover and regional muscle kinetics. *J. Am. Soc. Nephrol.*, 2005; 16, 862–868.

Ling, PR; Smith, RJ; Kie, S; et al. Effects of protein malnutrition on IL-6-mediated signaling in the liver and the systemic acute-phase response in rats. *Am. J. Physiol. Regul. Integr Comp. Physiol*, 2004; 287, 801–808.

Locatelli, F; Fouque, D; Heimburger, O; Drueke, TB; Cannata-Andia, JB; Horl, WH; et al. Nutritional status in dialysis patients: a European consensus. *Nephrol. Dial Transplant.*, 2002; 17(4), 563-72.

Lu, L; Erhard, P; Salomon, RG; Weiss, MF. Serum Vitamin E and Oxidative Protein Modification in Hemodialysis: A Randomized Clinical Trial. *American Journal of Kidney Diseases,* 2007; 50(2), 305-313.

Mafra, D; Cozzolino, SMF. Zinco protoporfirina como parâmetro de deficiência de ferro na insuficiência renal crônica. *J. Bras Nefrol.*, 2000; 22, 152-6.

Mahesh, S; Kaskel, F. Growth hormone axis in chronic kidney disease. *Pediatr. Nephrol.*, 2008; 23, 41-8.

Mak, RHK; DeFronzo. RA. Glucose and insulin metabolism in uremia. *Nephron.*, 1992; 61, 377–382.

Mak, RH. Insulin resistance but IGF-I sensitivity in chronic renal failure. *Am. J. Physiol.* 1996; 271, 114–119.

Mak, RH; Cheung, W; Cone, RD; et al. Leptin and inflammation- associated cachexia in chronic kidney disease. *Kidney Int*, 2006; 69, 794-797.

Martins, C; Cuppari, L; Avesani, C; Gusmão, MG. Terapia Nutricional para Pacientes em Hemodiálise Crônica - Projeto Diretrizes. Associação Médica Brasileira e Conselho Federal de Medicina. *Revista da Sociedade Brasileira de Nutrição Parenteral e Enteral,* 2011.

Massy, ZA; Nguyen-Khoa, T. Oxidative stress and chronic renal failure: markers and management. *J. Nephrol*, 2002; 15, 336–341.

Mehrotra, R; Kopple, JD; Wolfson, M. Metabolic acidosis in maintenance dialysis patients: clinical considerations. *Kidney Int.*, 2003; 64(88), S13-S25.

Mitch, WE; Du, J; Bailey, JL; Price, SR. Mechanisms causing muscle proteolysis in uremia: the influence of insulin and cytokines. *Miner. Electrolyte Metab.*, 1999; 25(4-6), 216-19.

Mitch, WE. Insights into the abnormalities of chronic renal disease attributed to malnutrition. *J. Am. Soc. Nephrol.*, 2002; 13(Suppl. 1), S22-S27.

Mitchell, ME. Carnitine metabolism in humans subjects. II. Values of carnitine in biological fluids and tissues of "normal" subjects. *Am. J. Clin. Nutr.*, 1978; 31(3), 481-91.

Moyle, GJ; Daar, ES; Gertner, JM; et al. Growth hormone improves lean body mass, physical performance, and quality of life in subjects with HIV-associated weight loss or wasting on highly active antiretroviral therapy. *J. Acquir. Immune Defic. Syndr.*, 2004; 35, 367–375.

National Kidney Foundation. K/DOQI clinical practice guidelines for chronic kidney disease: evaluation, classification, and stratification. *Am. J. Kidney Dis.*, 2002; 39(2 Suppl 1), S1-266.

Om, P; Hohenegger, M. Energy metabolism in acute uremic rats. *Nephron.*, 1980; 25(5), 249-53.

O'Sullivan, AJ; Lawson, JA; Chan, M; Kelly, JJ. Body composition and energy metabolism in chronic renal insufficiency. *Am. J. Kidney Dis.*, 2002; 39(2), 369-75.

Panesar, A; Agarwal, R. Resting energy expenditurein chronic kidney disease: relationship with glomerular filtration rate. *Clin. Nephrol.*, 2003; 59(5), 360-6.

Papagianni, A; Kalovoulos, M; Kirmizis, D; Vainas, A; Belechri, AM; Alexopoulos, E; et al. Carotid atherosclerosis is associated with inflammation and endothelial cell adhesion molecules in chronic haemodialysis patients. *Nephrol. Dial Transplant*. 2003; 18(1), 113-9.

Parfrey, PS; Foley, RN. The clinical epidemiology of cardiac disease in chronic renal failure. *J. Am. Soc. Nephrol.*, 1999; 10, 1606–1615.

Pupim, LB; Cuppari, L; Ikizler, TA. Nutrition and metabolism in kidney disease. *Semin. Nephrol.*, 2006; 26(2), 134-57.

Rammohan, M; Kalantar-Zadeh, K; Liang, A; et al. Megestrol acetate in a moderate dose for the treatment of malnutritioninflammation complex in maintenance dialysis patients. *J. Ren. Nutr.* 2005; 15, 345-355.

Remer, T. Influence of nutrition on acid-base balance. *Eur. J. Nutr.*. 2001; 40(5), 214-20.

Reuter, SE; Faull, RJ; Evans, AM. L-carnitine supplementation in the dialysis population—are Australian patients missing out? *Nephrology*, 2007; 13, 3–16.

Roob, JM; Khoschsorur, G; Tiran, A; Horina, JH; Holzer, H; Winklhofer-Roob B. Vitamin E attenuates oxidative stress induced by intravenous iron in patients on hemodialysis. *Jam. Soc. Nephrol*, 2000; 11, 539-549.

Ross, R. Atherosclerosis - an inflammatory disease. *N Engl J Med.*, 1999; 340(2), 115-26.

Samuelsson, O; Attman, PO; Knight Gibson, C; Kron, B. et al. Lipoprotein abnormalities without hyperlipidaemia in moderate renal insufficiency. *Nephrol. Dial. Transplant.*, 1991; 9, 1580-1585.

Schmid, DA; Held, K; Ising, M; et al. Ghrelin stimulates appetite. imagination of food, GH, ACTH, and cortisol, but does not affect leptin in normal controls. *Neuropsychopharmacology*, 2005; 30, 1187-1192.

Schneeweiss, B; Graninger, W; Stockenhuber, F; et al. Energy metabolism in acute and chronic renal failure. *Am. J. Clin. Nutr.*, 1990; 52, 596–601.

Selvin, E; Erlinger, TP. Prevalence of and risk factors for peripheral arterial disease in the United States: results from the National Health and Nutrition Examination Survey, 1999-2000. *Circulation*, 2004; 110, 738-43.

Shlipak, MG; Fried, LF; Cushman, M; Manolio, TA; Peterson, D; Stehman- Breen, C; et al. Cardiovascular mortality risk in chronic kidney disease: comparison of traditional and novel risk factors. *JAMA*. 2005; 293(14), 1737-45.

Silva, P. Renal fuel utilization, energy requirements, and function. *Kidney Int.*, 1987; 32(Suppl 22), 9-14.

Slatopolsky, E; Bricker, NS. The role of phosphorus restriction in the prevention of secondary hyperparathyroidism in chronic renal diseases. *Kidney Int*, 1993; 4, 141-5.

Sotirakopoulos, N; Athanasiou, G; Tsitsios, T; et al. Effect of L-carnitine supplementation on red blood cells deformability in hemodialysis patients. *Ren. Fail*, 2000; 22, 73–80.

Steiber, AL; Kopple, JD. Vitamin Status and Needs for People with Stages 3-5 Chronic Kidney Disease. *Journal of Renal Nutrition*, 2011; 21 (5), 355-368.

Stenvinkel, P; Heimburger, O; Lindholm, B; Kaysen, GA; Bergstrom, J. Are there two types of malnutrition in chronic renal failure? Evidence for relationships between malnutrition, inflammation and atherosclerosis (MIA syndrome). *Nephrol Dial Transplant.*, 2000; 15(7), 953-60.

Stenvinkel, P. Inflammation in end-stage renal disease—a fire that burns within. *Contrib. Nephrol*, 2005; 149, 185–199.

Stenvinkel, P. Inflammation in end-stage renal disease: the hidden enemy. *Nephrology*. 2006; 11(1), 36-41.

Suki, W.N.; Rouse, D. Renal transport of calcium, magnesium and phosphorus. In: Brenner, B.M. *The Kidney*. 4th ed., W.B. Saunders: Philadelphia; 1991; p.841-887.

Szeto, CC; Chow, KM. Metabolic acidosis and malnutrition in dialysis patients. *Semin. Dial.*, 2004; 17(5), 371-5.

Tomson, CR. Advising dialysis patients to restrict fluid intake without restricting sodium intake is not based on evidence and is a waste of time. *Nephrol. Dial Transplant*, 2001; 16, 1538 – 1542.

Tonelli, M; Bohm, C; Pandeya, S; Gill, J; Levin, A; Kiberd, BA. Cardiac risk factors and the use of cardioprotective medications in patients with chronic renal insufficiency. *Am. J. Kidney Dis.*, 2001; 37, 484-9.

Ulinski, T; Cochat, P. Longitudinal growth in children following kidney transplantation: from conservative to pharmacological strategies. *Pediatr. Nephrol.*, 2006; 21, 903-9.

Valderrábano, F; Jofre, R; López-Gómez, JM. Quality of life in end-stage renal disease patients. *Am. J. Kidney Dis.*, 2001; 38(3), 443-64.

Van Der Sluis, IM; Boot, AM; Nauta, J; et al. Bone density and body composition in chronic renal failure: effects of growth hormone treatment. *Pediatr. Nephrol*, 2000; 15, 221–228.

Van Vlen, B; Schoonjans, R; Vanholder, R; Vandamme, W; De Vos, M; Lameire, N. Dyspepsia and gastric emptying in chronic renal failure patients. *Clin. Nephrol.* 2001; 56(4), 302-7.

Vesel´a, E; Racek, J; Trefil, L; et al. Effect of L-carnitine supplementation in hemodialysis patients. *Nephron*, 2001; 88, 218–223.

Vimalanchandra, D; Hodson, EM; Willis, NS; Craig, JC; Cowell, C; Knight, JF. Growth hormone for children with chronic kidney disease (Cochrane Review). *Cochrane Database Syst Rev.*, 2006; doi: 10.1002/14651858.CD003264.

Vinuesa, SG; Ortega, M; Martinez, P; Goicoechea, M; Campdera, FG; Luno, J. Subclinical peripheral arterial disease in patients with chronic kidney disease: prevalence and related risk factors. *Kidney Int Suppl.* 2005; 93, S44-7.

Zima, T; Stipek, S; Crkovska, J; Nemecek, K; Platenik, K; Bartova, V; Tesar, V. Antioxidant enzymes: superoxide dismutase and glutathione peroxidade in haemodialysed patients. *Blood Purif*, 1996; 14, 257-61.

Wiggins, KL; Harvey, KS. A Review of Guidelines for Nutrition Care of Renal Patients. *Journal of Renal Nutrition*, 2002; 12 (3), 190-196.

Williams, R. Growth hormone underutilized in pediatric hemodialysis population. *Nat. Clin. Pract. Nephrol.*, 2006; 2(2), doi:10.1038/ncpneph0081.

Wiseman, AC; Linas, S. Disorders of potassium and acid-base balance. *Am. J. Kidney Dis.*, 2005; 45(5), 941-9.

Wynne, K; Stanley, S; McGowan, B; et al. Appetite control. *J. Endocrinol*, 2005; 184, 291-318.

In: Hemodialysis: Indications, Procedures and Complications ISBN: 978-1-62081-301-0
Editors: Y F. Cabral and M. Costa De Santos

Chapter III

Hemodialysis: Indications, Vascular Access, Different Modalities and Complications

Robert Ekart[1] and Radovan Hojs[2]
Clinic for Internal Medicine
[1]Department of Dialysis
and [2]Department of Nephrology,
University Medical Centre Maribor, Slovenia

Abstract

Despite the widespread use of peritoneal dialysis and renal transplantation, hemodialysis remains the main renal replacement therapy in most countries worldwide. Hemodialysis is required in three general situations: acute renal failure, end-stage renal disease and poisonings. Successful hemodialysis in any of these settings requires access to large blood vessels capable of supporting rapid extracorporeal blood flow. Central venous catheters are the preffered vascular access for patients presenting with acute renal failure and for chronic end-stage renal disease patients without permanent arteriovenous access or with failed vascular access. Adequate and timely preparation of vascular access in patients with chronic kidney disease stage 4 (estimated glomerular filtration rate below 30 ml per min per 1,73 m^2) can decrease morbidity and perhaps mortality. The access should generally be placed in the nondominant upper extremity. Venipuncture should therefore be restricted to the arm not chosen for eventual access placement so that the veins in the other arm will be preserve. There are a number of clinical indications to initiate dialysis in patients with acute renal failure or end-stage renal disease. These include: pericarditis or pleuritis (urgent indication), progressive uremic encephalopathy or neuropathy, with signs such as confusion, asterixis, tremor, multifocal myoclonus, wrist or foot drop, or, in severe cases, seizures (urgent indication), a clinically significant bleeding diathesis attributable to uremia (urgent indication), fluid overload refractory to diuretics, hypertension poorly responsive to antihypertensive medications, persistent metabolic disturbances that are refractory to medical therapy - hyperkalemia, metabolic acidosis, hypercalcemia, hypocalcemia, and hyperphosphatemia, persistent nausea and vomiting, evidence of malnutrition. Relative indications for the initiation of dialysis include decreased attentiveness and cognitive tasking, depression, persistent pruritus or the restless leg syndrome. Usually dialysis is initiated in adult patients with chronic kidney disease when the estimated glomerular filtration rate decrease to about 10 mL per minute per 1.73 m^2.

Multiple modalities of renal replacement therapy are currently available. These include intermittent hemodialysis, hemofiltration and hemodiafiltration, continuous renal replacement therapies, and hybrid therapies, such as sustained low-efficiency dialysis. Continuous renal replacement therapies represents a family of continuous modalities that provide support for severely ill patients with acute renal failure.

The most common acute complications during hemodialysis treatments are hypotension, hypertension, cramps, nausea and vomiting, headache, chest pain, back pain, itching. These complications are generally caused by multiple underlying mechanisms and are poorly understood.

This chapter will review indications, vascular access, different modalities and common and less common complications in patients undergoing hemodialysis treatment.

Introduction

For more than 2 million patients in the world who have reached end stage renal disease (ESRD), hemodialysis has become a routine therapy. It should not be forgotten that this life-saving treatment has only been routinely applied for ESRD for the past 40 years. The highest prevalence for ESRD is found in Japan at 2045 per million population, followed then by United States with a rate of 1509 per million population.

The worldwide prevalence rates of ESRD varies greatly, with less than 10 per million population reported by several countries. Currently, 52% of the global dialysis population resides in just four countries (United States, Japan, Germany, and Brazil) that make up only 11% of the world population. The reasons for the broad ranges of reported ESRD prevalence are likely wide difference in access to treatment, the availability of specific modalities of therapy, and methods of reimbursement between nations.

Input from a nephrologist should be obtained once chronic kidney disease (CKD) has been identified. The frequency of visits will increase as renal function declines. Once a patient has reached stage 4 CKD (estimated glomerular filtration rate (eGFR) of < 30 ml per minute per 1,73m^2), ideally he or she is under a nephrologist´s care every 3 months, and the risk factors associated with cardiovascular disease and progression are being optimally managed.

There is evidence that referral to nephrologist influence the time at which dialysis is initiated and subsequent outcome.

Survival of ESRD patients on dialysis depends to a large extent on their condition at the time dialysis was first initiated. It is important to pay attention to control of blood pressure, anemia, calcium/phosphorus intake, and nutrition during the predialysis period, as is timely insertion of arteriovenous fistula if hemodialysis has been selected.

When this is done using a multidisciplinary predialysis education program that include patient and family education, early choice of appropriate modality, and elective creation of dialysis access, the advantages have been fewer urgent dialyses, fewer hospital days in the first month after beginning dialysis, and substantial cost savings per patient at the time of commencing dialysis.

Initiation of Dialysis

Choice of Modality

1. Transplantation: It offers survival superior to the standard forms of dialysis being offered today. Transplantation may not be indicated for a patient who has severe problems with compliance in terms of medications.
2. Dialysis: Home versus in-center therapy: Among the ESRD therapies, the choices made will depend on what is available in the local community. One of the main decisions to be made is whether the patient will be coming in to a clinic for regular hemodialysis or whether the patient would prefer the independence of dialyzing at home, using either a home hemodialysis system or peritoneal dialysis. Transportation issues are very important here, as is the status of a patient´s home, the amount of support available through interested family members who might assist as caregivers, and technical issues such as available water quality and electricity.
3. Short daily hemodialysis: Whether done home or in-center, hemodialysis therapy is offered three times per week, usually 3-5 hours per session.
4. Long nocturnal hemodialysis: The nocturnal dialysis sessions are usually 8-10 hours in length. When given every other night, a therapy that can be delivered either at home or in-center, the weekly dialysis time is about 30 hours, compared to 12 hours in a usual three sessions x 4 hours dialysis schedule. Most patients on nocturnal hemodialysis dialyze 5-6 nights per week, giving 40-50 hours of treatment per week.
5. Peritoneal dialysis: Due to its simplicity, peritoneal dialysis offers patients a home-based therapy with very little requirement for special water systems and simple equipment setup time. There are two types of peritoneal dialysis for a patient to consider: continuous ambulatory peritoneal dialysis, where a patient performs manual exchanges four or five times per day, and automated peritoneal dialysis, where a patient hooks up to machine at night and exchanges are carried out automatically while the patient sleeps. Patients for whom peritoneal dialysis is often favored are: infants or very young children, patients with severe cardiovascular disease, patients with difficult vascular access, patients who desire greater freedom to travel. Contraindications to peritoneal dialysis include an unsuitable peritoneum due to presence of adhesions, fibrosis, or malignancy. Peritoneal dialysis allows patients independence and freedom to travel and does not constrain patients to a fixed in-center dialysis schedule.
6. The option not to dialyze: Palliative care. There are no absolute contraindications to dialysis therapy. Patient with advanced disease in an organ system other than the kidneys, or those with malignancy, have sometimes been excluded from chronic dialysis. Futility is an ethical principle on which one can make a reasonable decision not to initiate dialysis.

7. Elderly patients and dialysis: Patients older than 75-80 years are the fastest growing age group presenting for dialysis. Many elderly patients placed on dialysis continue to enjoy a good quality-of-life and benefit from documented improvement in a variety of health outcome measures.

Indication for Hemodialysis

The common indications for initiation of hemodialysis in patients with acute kidney failure include:

- pulmonary edema,
- refractory fluid overload,
- uncontrolled hypertension,
- metabolic acidosis (pH less than 7.1),
- hyperkalemia(plasma potassium concentration > 6.5 meq/L) or rapidly rising potassium levels,
- symptoms of uremia, such as nausea, vomiting, loose of appetite, fatigue, feeling of weakness and/or coldness, otherwise unexplained alteration in mental status (at first, only subtle changes in personality, but eventually, the patients become confused and comatose),
- signs of uremia, such as pericardial friction rub or evidence of pericardial effusion with or without tamponade, sallow coloration of the skin due to accumulation of urochrome pigment, uremic motor neuropathy (foot- or wrist-drop), uremic encephalopathy (tremor, asterixis, multifocal myoclonus, or seizures), prolongation of bleeding time.

The common indications for initiation of hemodialysis in patients with chronic kidney failure:

Usually dialysis is initiated in adult patients when the eGFR decrease to about 10 ml per minute per 1.73 m^2.However, evaluation of the need for dialysis should begin at a higher eGFR level, probably somewhere between 15 and 20 ml per minute per 1.73 m^2. Once the eGFR falls below 20 ml per minute per 1.73 m^2, patients should be periodically questioned regarding symptoms related to nutrition: loss of appetite, nausea and/or vomiting, especially in the morning owing to overnight retention of uremic toxins in the gut, and unintended weight loss. These are very often the earliest markers of uremia.

Certain patients, especially those with comorbidities, appear to be especially susceptible and may require earlier initiation of chronic dialysis, for example patients with advanced age and cognitive impairment, patients with advanced cardiac disease. It should be noted that pericarditis or pleuritis without other cause is an indication for urgent dialysis, particularly pericarditis, where the risk of rapidly developing pericardial effusion and cardiac tamponade is present.

Multiple lines of evidence suggest that the patient´s health status at the time of initiation of dialysis will affect subsequent morbidity and mortality. Protein intake often falls spontaneously as renal function deteriorates. This can lead to a loss of muscle mass and lower serum albumin levels. Cardiovascular diseases, the cause of the greatest mortality in the hemodialysis population, most often have their origin long before dialysis is initiated. Untreated or inadequately treated anemia may lead to worsened left ventricular hypertrophy and exacerbation of angina as the patient approaches ESRD.

Vascular Access for Hemodialysis

There are three major types of vascular access for maintenance hemodialysis: primary arteriovenous (AV) fistulas; synthetic arteriovenous fistulas (AV grafts); and tunneled and nontunneled central venous catheters.

The necessity for vascular access in patients with renal failure can be temporary or permanent. Temporary access is established by the percutaneous insertion of a catheter into a large vein (internal jugular, femoral, or, less desirably, subclavian). Construction of an ideal permanent vascular access delivers a flow adequate for the dialysis prescription, lasts a long time (months to years), and has a low complication rate.

It is important to identify patients who may eventually require renal replacement therapy since adequate preparation can decrease morbidity and perhaps mortality. Early identification enables dialysis to be initiated at the optimal time with a functioning chronic access. The maintenance of adequate, durable vascular access for hemodialysis is essential for the well-being of the patient with ESRD. The provision of hemodialysis requires repeated vascular access that can achieve a blood flow in excess of 350 ml/min. The access should generally be placed in the nondominant upper extremity, because of the increased risk of infection and more severe consequences of arterial steal syndrome with lower extremity grafts. Venipuncture should therefore be restricted to the arm not chosen for eventual access placement so that the veins in the other arm will be preserved. Since a primary AV fistula requires months to mature and is the access of choice, patients should be referred for surgery to attempt access construction when it is estimated that the patient is within one year of the anticipated need for dialysis as manifested by eGFR less than 25 mL/min, a plasma creatinine concentration greater than 4 mg/mL (354 micromol/L), or a rapid rate of progression. The 2006 K/DOQI guidelines recommend that a fistula be placed at least six months prior to the anticipated start of hemodialysis.

Preoperative evaluation: A thorough history is required, querying about previous episodes of central vein cannulations or intravenous pacemaker implantation, prior use of percutaneously inserted central catheter lines, stroke, smoking, amputation or prior additional vascular surgery. Comorbid conditions such as congestive heart failure, diabetes mellitus, or peripheral vascular disease may limit options for access construction. The major contraindication to creation of any AV access is advanced calcifying arteriosclerosis. Patients with severe heart failure may not tolerate the additional cardiac output required to circulate blood through the access. Patients with severe vascular disease due to atherosclerosis or diabetes or patients with extensive damage to their arm veins due to prior needle sticks may not have adequate blood vessels to support creation of an AV access.

Physical examination with palpation of arterial pulses, and venous vasculature, an Allen test of radial and ulnar blood flow in both arms, and blood pressure measurement in both arms is required.

Routine preoperative maping of the arm to evaluate veins and arteries helps with selection of the most appropriate vein and the best location of the access. Doppler ultrasonography, which can measure flow velocity as well as the inner diameter of the brachial and radial arteries and peripheral veins, should be performed in all patients to detect central vein stenosis and to identify suitable arteries and veins for fistula or graft placement. The resistance index in the feeding artery lower than 0.7 indicates insufficient arterial compliance. Minimum size of the feeding artery for a successful fistula should be between 1.5 and 2.0 mm in diameter. The vein should be at least 2.5 mm in diameter at the point of anastomosis to increase AV fistula success.

Primary AV fistulas: Primary AV fistulas are the preferred form of vascular access given their significantly higher long-term patency rates and lower rate of complications. Creation of a native vein fistula requires that an anastomosis be made between an adequate artery and an adequate vein in close proximity to each other. At least nine potential sites for AV fistulas can be found in an upper extremity. The most commonly used site is at the wrist, where the cephalic vein is connected to the radial artery (Brescia-Cimino fistula). The original operation described by Brescia and colleagues was a side-to-side artery-to-vein anastomosis. However, the end-to-side configuration is preffered by many surgeons today as there is a lower incidence of venous hypertension in the hand. A well constructed radiocephalic fistula that functions for the first six months can be expected to function for up to 20 years.

Whereas radiocephalic fistulas are preffered when feasible, several reports suggest that when an aggressive approach is undertaken, a high percentage of radiocephalic fistulas either fail to mature or develop thrombosis. Failure of radiocephalic fistula maturation is especially prevalent in female, diabetic, and older hemodialysis patients.

An alternative to the radiocephalic fistula is to use the upper arm veins to create either a brachiocephalic fistula or a brachiobasilic fistula. Because the basilic vein in the upper arm generally lies under deep fascia, use of this vein for an AV fistula requires that the vein be dissected and transposed into a more convenient subcutaneous position. The brachial artery can also be anastomosed to a perforating vein, joining the superficial and deep venous system just below the elbow crease (the Gracz fistula). Compared with brachiocephalic fistulas, transposed brachiobasilic fistulas are more likely to mature but have a higher long-term thrombosis rate.

Following surgery, the arm should initially be kept elevated and tight circumferential dressings should be avoided. The fistula blood flow should be checked daily. The fistula should never be used for venipuncture. Hand exercises may help increase blood flow and pressure, thereby accelerating maturation, the process which generally requires at least 4 weeks, but may require up to 6 months. At the time of intended use, the vein diameter should be at least 4 mm and blood flow at least 600 ml per minute.

Synthetic AV access (bridge grafts): An AV graft is a second-line access procedure when an AV fistula cannot be successfully constructed and maintained. The use of AV grafts as initial vascular access should be a very rare event. Nevertheless, AV grafts have some advantages, including an initial high blood flow rate, large surface area for needle placement, easy cannulation, first cannulation within 2 to 3 weeks, and, with special graft materials even a few days after insertion. Theoretically, AV grafts can be placed at any site between an artery and a vein, but excellent artery inflow and excellent venous outflow are prerequisites. AV grafts constructed with synthetic material, most commonly polytetrafluoroethylene (PTFE), provide excellent vascular access in patients who fail endogenous AV fistula placement. PTFE has good surgical handling characteristics, and grafts of this material usually mature in two weeks. Short grafts have no advantage over long grafts in terms of patency and longevity. The most common initial sites for AV graft placement are a straight graft from the radial artery at the wrist to the basilic vein; a loop graft in the forearm from the brachial artery to the basilic vein; or an upper arm graft from brachial artery to axillary vein. A distal graft in the nondominant arm is generally preferred initially. Synthetic grafts have a higher long-term complication rate (eg, infection, thrombosis) than primary fistulas. Unfortunately, the current 1- and 2-year primary patency rate for PTFE grafts are a dismal 50% and 25%, respectively. Graft thrombosis accounts for 80% of all vascular access dysfunction, and in over 90% of thrombosed grafts, venous stenosis is detected at or distal to the graft vein anastomosis. The underlying pathology for the development of venous stenosis is venous neointimal hyperplasia, neoangiogenesis within the neointima and adventitia. The 2006 K/DOQI guidelines recommend that a synthetic graft be placed at least three to six weeks prior to the anticipated start of hemodialysis. Complications related to AV vascular access are stenosis, thrombosis, ischemia in a limb bearing an AV access, pseudoaneurysm, infections, and congestive heart failure.

Central venous dialysis catheters: Dialysis catheters are a necessary evil, allowing dialysis in patients who do not have permanent AV access. They expose patients to a greater risk of complications compared to an AV fistula, including a five- to sevenfold increased risk of infection and in some studies an increase in mortality.

Short term venous catheters are commonly used for acute vascular access in the following patients:

- those with acute renal failure;
- those requiring hemodialysis or hemoperfusion for overdose or intoxication;
- those with ESRD needing urgent hemodialysis but without available mature access;
- those on maintenance hemodialysis who have lost effective use of their permanent access and require temporary access until permanent access function can be re-established;
- peritoneal dialysis patients whose abdomens are being rested prior to new peritoneal catheter placement;
- patients requiring plasmapheresis; and
- transplant recipients needing temporary hemodialysis during severe rejection episodes.

Temporary untunneled dialysis catheters can be inserted at the bedside using the modified Seldinger technique with only local anesthesia. Real-time ultrasound-guided venous puncture is recommended for catheter insertion. The optimal insertion site is the right internal jugular vein. The subclavian site should generally be avoided, as there is a significant risk of subsequent venous stenosis preventing the successful creation of a permanent vascular access. Catheterization of the femoral vein is a good choice when the need for hemodialysis or hemoperfusion or plasmapheresis is expected to be less than one week.

The femoral approach is useful for performing the initial hemodialysis treatment in patients who present with acute pulmonary oedema because the patient`s head and chest can be elevated during insertion.

Tunneled cuffed vascular catheters are inserted under fluoroscopic guidance, and the cuff, often made of Dacron, is positioned inside the skin tunnel allowing for fibroblast ingrowth and subsequently the risk of infection. This type of catheter is most commonly inserted in the right internal jugular vein and tunneled under the skin to the below the clavicle; however, they can be placed in any large vein if clinically indicated due to limited vascular access sites.

This type of catheter is appropriate for patients who are anticipated to require dialysis for more than 3 weeks, even if they have acute renal failure.

Long term vascular catheters are utilizied for patients in whom an AV access cannot be readily created. Such patients include small children, some diabetic patients, with severe vascular disease, patients who are morbidly obese, and patients who have undergone multiple AV access insertions and in whom additional sites for AV access insertion are not available. Additional indications include patients with cardiomyopathy unable to sustain adequate blood pressure or access flows.

Patients being dialyzed with venous catheters do not do as well as those using an AV access. Catheter patients develop infections more often, they have higher levels of inflammatory markers, and they die more frequently. It is unclear if these associative risks reflect a different patient population receiving catheters, some risk factor that occur when AV accesses fail and a catheter must be placed, or if they are due completely to some property of catheter use per se. Inadequate blood flow through catheters remains a significant problem.

Complications related to central venous catheterization are immediate (arterial puncture, pneumothorax, hemothorax, air embolism, arrhytmias, perforation of vein or cardiac chamber, pericardial tamponade), delayed (infection, thrombosis, vascular stricture, arteriovenous fistula) and injury to adjacent structures (trachea, brachial plexus, recurrent laryngeal nerve).

Different Modalities of Dialysis

The goal of hemodialysis in patients with ESRD is to restore the body`s intracellular and extracellular fluid environment toward the body composition of healthy individuals with functioning kidneys to the extent possible. Although the life expectancy of patients with ESRD has improved since the introduction of dialysis in the 1960s, it is still far below that of the general population. As an example, the mean life span at age 49 in the United States is 33 years in the general population but only approximately seven years in patients receiving maintenance dialysis, in whom the overall five-year survival rate is about 30 to 50 percent in nondiabetics (depending upon the diagnosis) and 25 percent in diabetics.

Previously, one partial explanation for the poor survival in the United States was inadequate dialysis, since substantially higher survival rates have been reported in Europe and Japan even after case adjustment for age, sex, and renal diagnoses.

Japanese patients, for example, have far fewer comorbid risk factors than those in the United States. However, it is more likely that factors such as older age, a higher prevalence of diabetes mellitus, and more comorbid conditions are components of the higher dialysis mortality in the United States. This is particularly true as an increasing dialysis dose has been realized in the United States. One of the highest survival rates has been reported from Tassin,

France where patients are dialyzed 24 hours per week, much longer than in almost all other centers. This and other observations has led to a general increase in time in the dialysis prescription in the United States.

Selection of Dialysis Modality

There are two principal choices for maintenance dialysis: hemodialysis and peritoneal dialysis. Selecting one of these modalities is influenced by a number of considerations such as availability and convenience, comorbid conditions, socioeconomic and dialysis center factors, the patient's home situation, method of physician reimbursement, and the ability to tolerate volume shifts. The percentage of patients undergoing hemodialysis far surpasses those being maintained on peritoneal dialysis. Based on the 2009 USRDS report, 94 and 6 percent respectively began hemodialysis and peritoneal dialysis in the United States, respectively. About 2.5 percent of patients with ESRD received a renal transplant as the initial treatment for their ESRD.

The use of hemodialysis as renal replacement therapy is accomplished via solute removal from the blood into the dialysate, as exemplified by intradialytic removal of potassium, urea, and phosphorous, as well as the addition of solute from the dialysate into the blood, as is exemplified by bicarbonate and calcium. An additional goal of the dialysis procedure is the elimination of excess water volume from the patient via ultrafiltration. Thus, the prescription for an individual hemodialysis session must take in to account an examination and physiologic assessment of individual patient needs in order to achieve these goals. The variables in the hemodialysis prescription that may be manipulated by the each physician on the basis of clinical assessment are time of dialysis, dialysis frequency, hemodialyzer, anticoagulation, blood flow rate, dialysate flow rate, ultrafiltration rate, dialysate temperature, dialysate composition and intradialytic medications.

The principles that underlie the hemodialysis procedure are simple in practice. Blood and dialysate are circulated on opposite sides of a semipermeable membrane, thereby permitting the passage of solutes elevated as a consequence of renal failure but restricting the transfer of blood proteins and cellular elements. The device containing the semipermeable membrane is the hemodialyzer. Removal of water occurs by control of the hydrostatic pressure gradient across the semipermeable membrane and may be augmented by increasing the osmolality of the dialysate fluid.

Hemofiltration differs markedly from hemodialysis by the mechanisms by which the composition of the blood is modified. During hemofiltration, the filtrate is discarded and the patient receives a substitution fluid either before (predilution) or after (postdilution) the hemodialyzer. The substitution fluid contains the major crystalloid components of the plasma at physiologic levels. Both bicarbonate and lactate are used as buffers. The rate of fluid removal and substitution fluid infusion can be adapted to the patient`s need. In patients with fluid overload, a negative fluid balance can be obtained by replacing less fluid through infusion that is removed. Hemofiltration is particulary useful as a continuous renal replacement therapy in an intensive care setting. The hemodynamic stability characteristic of convective therapies is confirmed also in comparison with modern hemodialysis.

Hemodiafiltration combines the benefits of hemodialysis (high transport rate of low molecular weight solutes by diffusion) and hemofiltration (high convective transport of substances). Hemodiafiltration is used both as a continuous and an intermittent renal replacement therapy. Hemodiafiltration offers a potential benefit regarding anemia correction, inflammation, lipid profiles, oxidative stress, and calcium – phosphate products and possibly the prevention of long term dialysis complications such as dialysis amyloidosis. Higher costs, and in some countries, the decisions of regulatory boards prevent the widespread use of hemodiafiltration, despite its likely benefits over conventional hemodialysis. Although virtually not used in the United States, hemodiafiltration is a form of chronic renal replacement therapy in Europe.

Adequacy of Hemodialysis

Hemodialysis needs to be prescribed and dosed according to the patients´s individual needs. From a clinical perspective, probably the best marker of adequacy is a physically active, well-nourished, nonanemic, normotensive patient with no compliants. Adequacy purely in terms of dialysis dose refers to delivery of a treatment dose that is considered high enough to promote an optimal long-term outcome.

Urea serves as surrogate marker for water soluble small molecular weight toxins, and in clinical practice, dialysis dose is expressed by urea reduction ratio or by the treatment index Kt/V. Simply following predialysis blood urea nitrogen levels is insufficient to assess dialysis dose because a low blood urea nitrogen may much reflect indaquate protein intake as a consequence of malnutrition rather than sufficient dialytic urea removal.

Dialyzers are highly efficient in removing urea from blood, reducing the urea concentration during one passage by 80% to 90%. During hemodialysis, the urea concentration in the blood compartment is always lower than in the tissue compartments. The urea rebound after hemodialysis is the period of equilibration between blood and tissue compartments and takes about 30 to 60 minutes. Urea reduction ratio is a simple but rather imprecise way to quantify dialysis dose and correlates well with dialysis outcome, and despite its limitations, it is an accepted method for assessment of dialysis adequacy. The treatment index Kt/V is the most widely used parameter to assess dialysis dose. Kt/V may be applies to any substance but in clinical practice is almost exclusively used for urea, where K is defined as the whole-body clearance rate for urea, t as the effective treatment time, and V as the body´s urea distribution volume (which equates closely to total body water). Other measures of urea removal are single-pool Kt/V, equilibrated Kt/V, and the weekly standard Kt/V.

The minimally adequate dose of hemodialysis given 3 times per week to patients with Kr (average of urea and creatinine clearances) less than 2 mL per min per 1.73 m^2 should be an single pool Kt/V of 1.2 per dialysis. For treatment times less than 5 hours, an alternative minimum dose is a urea reduction ratio of 65%. Efforts should be made to monitor and minimize the occurrence of missed or shortened treatments.

Home, Nocturnal, and Short-Daily Hemodialysis

Survival is generally highest in patients treated with home hemodialysis: up to 89 percent at five years, 74 percent at 15 years in nondiabetics, and 50 percent at 15 years overall. Despite this apparent advantage, the absolute number and relative percentage of patients with

ESRD who use home hemodialysis in the United States has slowly declined over the last decade and is much lower than that in some other countries. Nocturnal hemodialysis (eg, long-nightly-home hemodialysis, a form of quotidian hemodialysis) was introduced, principally in Canada, as a (possibly) more desirable alternative to conventional dialysis, since it provides superior dialysis based upon dose, duration, and frequency. This can be accomplished because it is performed during nightly sleep, an otherwise unproductive time.

Based on better outcomes in many biochemical areas, quality of life issues, blood pressure control, regression of left ventricular hypertrophy, improved sleep patterns and improved general well being, one would expect improved survival rates of these patients. There now are data suggesting that survival is truly improved with these modalities with lower mortalities and similar survival rates to deceased donor renal transplants. For all these reasons, nocturnal hemodialysis will be associated with improved patient survival since it provides the best clearance of uremic products along with remarkable hemodynamic stability (with only gradual changes in physiological parameters), and improved cardiovascular function with regression of left ventricular hypertrophy. Another modality is short hours high efficiency daily hemodialysis (another form of quotidian hemodialysis). This consists of hemodialysis occurring 5 to 6 days/week with a total duration of 1.5 to 2.5 hours per day. There is a paucity of data related to morbidity and/or mortality associated with this procedure.

Complications

Acute complications commonly occur during routine hemodialysis treatments. They include the following:

- Hypotension
- Hypertension
- Cramps
- Nausea and vomiting
- Headache
- Chest pain
- Itching

These complications are generally caused by multiple underlying mechanisms and are poorly understood. Knowledge of their pathogenesis is further complicated by their often simultaneous occurrence. As an example, hypotension with hemodialysis, which has a myriad of possible causes, may be accompanied by nausea, vomiting, headache, and/or chest pain. Similarly, cramps may be associated with hypotension and are often very difficult to treat.

Hypotension

The usual manifestation of hemodynamic instability during ultrafiltration dialysis is hypotension. The incidence of a symptomatic reduction in blood pressure during (or immediately following) dialysis ranges from 15 to 50 percent of dialysis sessions. In some patients, the development of orthostatic hypotension necessitates intravenous fluid replacement before they are able to leave the dialysis unit. This problem contributes to the excessive morbidity that is associated with the dialysis procedure.

There are two clinical patterns of dialysis-associated hypotension:

- Episodic hypotension, which typically occurs during the latter stages of dialysis; this is associated with vomiting, muscle cramps, and other vagal symptoms (such as yawning).
- Chronic persistent hypotension, which may occur in long-term patients in whom predialysis systolic blood pressures of less than 100 mmHg are frequently observed.

Although hypotension during hemodialysis is a frequent complication, some patients develop paradoxical hypertension in the later stages of dialysis.

Etiology of Hypotension

Many factors may contribute to dialysis hypotension, these include:

- Rapid fluid removal in an attempt to attain "dry weight", particularly among those with large interdialytic weight gains.
- Inaccurate determination of true "dry weight".
- A rapid reduction in plasma osmolality, which causes extracellular water to move into the cells.
- Autonomic neuropathy.
- Diminished cardiac reserve.
- Intake of antihypertensive medications that can impair cardiovascular stability. Use of a lower sodium concentration in the dialysate.
- Ingestion of a meal immediately before or during dialysis.
- Arrhythmias or pericardial effusion with tamponade, which are volume-unresponsive causes of hypotension.
- Reactions to the dialyzer membrane, which may cause wheezing and dyspnea as well as hypotension. Increased synthesis of endogenous vasodilators, such as nitric oxide.

Infrequently, patients with dialysis-induced hypotension have a serious medical condition requiring immediate attention. These include arrhythmias, pericardial tamponade, valvular disorders, myocardial infarction, hemolysis, hemorrhage, septicemia, and air embolism. Whatever the underlying cause, patients with hemodialysis-associated hypotension have increased mortality and morbidity. Patients with frequent intradialytic hypotension are at increased risk of fistula thrombosis. The overall rate of thrombosis was much higher among patients with grafts compared with AV fistulas.

Diagnosis and Treatment

Although occasionally asymptomatic, patients with hypotension may suffer from light-headedness, muscle cramps, nausea, vomiting, and dyspnea. The acute management of low blood pressure associated with hemodialysis includes the following:

- Ultrafiltration should either be stopped or the rate decreased.
- The patient should be placed in the Trendelenburg position.

- The blood flow rate should be reduced.
- Intravascular volume may be replaced with mannitol or intravenous bolus of saline.

Further treatment is based upon the etiology of the hypotension; the prompt recognition of life-threatening causes of low blood pressure is essential. Particular concerns should include occult sepsis, previously unrecognized cardiac and/or pericardial disease, and gastrointestinal bleeding. Patients with chronic, debilitating hemodialysis hypotension due to the inability to adequately respond to rapid changes in blood volume may be more likely to tolerate the gradual volume changes associated with peritoneal dialysis or nocturnal hemodialysis. Increasing the time and/or frequency of hemodialysis is another possibility.

Prevention of Hypotension

Moderate success can be achieved with therapies aimed at reducing the incidence of symptomatic dialysis hypotension. Among those with proven efficacy, the following appear to be the most beneficial in the patient undergoing maintenance hemodialysis:

Accurate Setting of the "Dry Weight"

At present, the determination of dry weight is largely determined empirically by trial and error. The dry weight is set at the weight below which unacceptable symptoms, such as cramping, nausea, and vomiting, or hypotension occur. The dry weight is highly variable in many patients, and can fluctuate with intercurrent illnesses (such as diarrhea or infection) and with changes in hemoglobin (as with erythropoietin). A large number of other modalities have been evaluated in an effort to more objectively estimate dry weight. These include blood volume monitoring, ultrasound assessment of the inferior vena cava, natriuretic peptide measurements, extravascular lung water indices, and bioimpedance methods. The best comparative studies have generally favored methods that rely upon bioimpedance measurements. These provide an assessment of extracellular and intracellular volume and total body water. Particular promise lies in a technique in which continuous intradialytic measurements are confined to the calf since the relative volume of excess extracellular fluids is greater in the lower extremities.

Steady, Constant Ultrafiltration

Some dialysis machines are equipped with accurate ultrafiltration devices that remove volume steadily and evenly over the course of the dialysis session. This has enabled patients to tolerate the procedure with fewer adverse events. Some physicians have advocated the use of modeling protocols in which more (or less) weight is removed at the beginning or end of dialysis. The efficacy of ultrafiltration/sodium modeling has not been proven, but it may help in selected cases. Increased weight loss has traditionally occurred in the setting of a higher dialysate sodium concentration.

Increased Dialysate Sodium Concentration and Sodium Modeling

The use of a higher dialysate sodium concentration ($\geq$140 meq/L) has been among the most efficacious and best tolerated therapies for episodic hypotension. The high sodium concentration prevents a marked decline in plasma osmolality during dialysis, thereby protecting the extracellular volume by minimizing osmotic fluid loss into the cells.

Combination Sodium Modeling and Ultrafiltration

Ultrafiltration profiling is characterized by the ultrafiltration rate being intermittently stopped or decreased gradually, thereby resulting in plasma refilling. The combination of ultrafiltration and sodium profiling can further enhance plasma refilling; in turn, this can result in greater stability during hemodialysis.

Temperature Control

The use of low dialysate temperature can improve hemodynamic stability by improving cardiovascular contractility and increasing venous tone. During standard hemodialysis, an increase in core temperature is commonly observed, with the underlying causes being ultrafiltration and several other factors. Isothermic dialysis, in which body temperature remains constant during the hemodialysis procedure, may prove useful in stabilizing blood pressure among hypotension-prone patients.

Hypertension

Hypertension is common in hemodialysis patients with major implications for survival. Using various definitions of hypertension, the prevalence of hypertension in hemodialysis patients is up to 90%. The diagnosis is often complicated especially because there are large swings in blood pressure with hemodialysis and it is difficult to accurately ascertain the blood pressure in the interdialytic period. The pathogenesis of hypertension in hemodialysis patients is multilayered and at present still not completely elucidated. One or more of the factors play a role in a individual patient – hypervolemia, increased sympathetic activity, erythropoietin, altered endotelial cell function and many others. The influence of hypertension on cardiovascular outcomes in hemodialysis patients is less clear, and complicated because of the high prevalence of comorbid conditions in these patients. Accurate measure of blood pressure is an essential precursor for management. Pre- and post-dialysis blood pressure measurement may not reflect the average blood pressure experienced by the patient. Most management decisions for the diagnosis and treatment of hypertension are made using blood pressure measurements made in the dialysis center. However, ambulatory blood pressure monitoring (ABPM) and home blood pressure recordings may be of superior prognostic value. They are generally superior to the dialysis center blood pressure measurements in predicting long-term prognosis. In addition, ABPM and home blood pressure recordings significantly and strongly predict cardiovascular events. The reference standard for diagnosing hypertension among hemodialysis patients is 44-48 hour interdialytic ABPM. Hypervolemia that is not clinically obvious is the most common treatable cause of hypertension among patients with ESRD; thus, volume control should be the initial therapy to treat hypertension in most hemodialysis patients. Reducing dietary and dialysate sodium is an often overlooked strategy to improve blood pressure control. The treatment should be guided by blood pressure obtained outside the dialysis center. In general, all antihypertensive drugs can be used in the hemodialysis population with doses determined by dialyzability and hemodynamic instability. Renin-angiotensin-aldosterone system inhibitors have been shown to improve cardiovascular morbidity and mortality and are recommended as the initial pharmacologic therapy for hypertensive hemodialysis patients.

Muscle Cramps

Muscle cramps are a common complication of hemodialysis treatments; they often result in the early termination of a hemodialysis session and are therefore a significant cause of underdialysis. The exact etiology of cramps in dialysis patients is unknown. Since cramps tend to occur most frequently near the end of hemodialysis treatments, changes in plasma osmolality and/or extracellular fluid volume have been implicated.

A cramp is a prolonged involuntary muscle contraction that occurs in a muscle which voluntarily contracts when it is already in its most shortened position. The etiology of hemodialysis-associated cramps may include contributions from one or more of the following factors: plasma volume contraction, hyponatremia, tissue hypoxia, hypomagnesemia. Of these, volume contraction and hyponatremia, either alone or in combination, are the most likely underlying causative factors; this hypothesis is supported in part by the reduction in the frequency of cramping in association with sodium modeling or ramping, a technique whereby gradual decrements in dialysate sodium concentration occur over the course of a hemodialysis treatment.

Cramps occurring with hemodialysis treatment most commonly involve the muscles of the lower extremity, but the muscles of the hands, arms, and abdomen may also be affected. Cramps occur more often in older, nondiabetic, anxious patients. Low parathyroid hormone values and high serum creatine phosphokinase concentrations are also more frequent among patients with dialysis-associated cramps. Multiple factors related to the dialysis procedure enhance the risk of cramps are solute concentrations of the dialysate bath, particularly low concentrations of sodium and increased ultrafiltration required to remove excessive fluid ingested in the interdialytic period.

Treatment is directed at two goals: reducing the frequency of cramps and relieving symptoms when they occur. The minimization of interdialytic weight gains, the prevention of dialysis-associated hypotension, the use of high concentrations of sodium in the dialysate, and carnitine supplementation may all reduce the frequency of dialysis-associated cramps. Minimizing interdialytic weight gains will avoid plasma volume contraction and hypoosmolality that occurs with high rates of ultrafiltration required to achieve the patient's dry weight during a brief dialysis session; such measures may prevent or at least reduce the frequency of dialysis-associated cramps.

The reversal of low blood pressure should be the first priority in the management of the patient with muscle cramps in association with hypotension. If necessary, ultrafiltration should either be stopped or the rate decreased, the patient should be placed in the Trendelenburg position, and the blood flow rate should be reduced. The clinician must also be aware that hypotension may be a manifestation of a potentially serious medical condition requiring immediate attention. Further measures to treat dialysis-associated cramps are generally aimed at increasing plasma osmolality.

A variety of additional medications and/or agents have been used to prevent leg cramps. They are of variable efficacy and have rarely been tested in controlled trials in either dialysis or non-ESRD populations.

These include short acting benzodiazepines (eg, oxazepam), nifedipine, phenytoin, creatine monohydrate, carbamazepine, amitriptyline, and gabapentin.

Headache, Nausea, and Vomiting

Longer treatment times and/or ultrafiltration in association with a large degree of solute removal significantly enhance the incidence of headache, nausea, and vomiting during hemodialysis.

It is important to emphasize that longer treatment times alone may not necessarily be associated with adverse effects. The lack of such effects with extended hemodialysis treatment times in the dialysis center in Tassin, France as well as with nocturnal hemodialysis indicate that length of treatment alone may be unimportant if the solute clearance rate is slow. In addition, dialyzer membrane composition, surface area, and biocompatibility are not significant factors underlying these intradialytic symptoms.

Since longer treatment times combined with high urea removal rates appear to be important, a variant of the dialysis disequilibrium syndrome may underlie these symptoms in many patients. Dialysis disequilibrium is thought to be due to water movement into the brain as a result of a reverse osmotic shift induced by urea removal.

Although quite uncommon, the syndrome should be considered in the noncompliant and/or inadequately dialyzed patient who develops nausea, vomiting, or headache while being aggressively dialyzed. In this setting, initially altering the dialysis prescription in favor of less intensive and more frequent treatments may avoid these complications. Patients who have headaches on dialysis in the absence of hypotension and suspected dialysis disequilibrium should be questioned about caffeine use, which can sometimes precipitate headache.

In addition, metabolic disturbances (eg, hypoglycemia, hypernatremia, and hyponatremia), uremia, subdural hematoma, and medication-induced headaches should be considered in patients with recurrent dialysis-associated headaches. Rarely, dialysis-associated headache may be associated with increased intra-ocular pressure. In some patients, psychological factors may contribute to dialysis-associated somatic complaints.

Chest Pain

Chest pain that occurs while a patient is being dialyzed may be associated with hypotension or dialysis disequilibrium syndrome. Additional possibilities should always be considered; these include angina pectoris, hemolysis, and (rarely) air embolism. Furthermore, although pulmonary embolism is extremely uncommon in dialysis patients, this complication may be observed after manipulation of thrombus and/or occlusion of the dialysis access. Acutely, the decision to continue or stop the dialysis treatment because of chest pain is based upon clinical findings, such as hemodynamic stability, and the results of the history and physical examination.

Angina pectoris should always be considered as the underlying cause of chest discomfort in the patient undergoing hemodialysis given the increased incidence of coronary disease in this setting. The appropriate history, physical examination, and, if clinically indicated, electrocardiogram and cardiac enzyme evaluation should therefore be performed. If hemodialysis is continued, the administration of oxygen and aspirin, reduction of the desired ultrafiltration and/or blood pump speed, and administration of nitrates or morphine should be considered on an individual basis. Angina pectoris during hemodialysis may be prevented with the administration of nitrates and/or beta blockers prior to the treatment. However, the efficacy of these agents is diminished since they commonly result in hypotension, thereby reducing the ability to effectively remove extracellular fluid.

Hemolysis may present as chest pain, chest tightness, or back pain. It deserves consideration as an etiologic factor in the patient with these complaints, particularly if multiple individuals have such symptoms simultaneously. If hemolysis is not recognized early, severe hyperkalemia may ensue and lead to death. Findings highly suggestive of substantial hemolysis include: a port wine appearance of the blood in the venous line, complaints of chest pain, shortness of breath, and/or back pain, a falling hematocrit, a pink color of the plasma in centrifuged specimens.

The etiology of hemolysis in hemodialysis patients is usually related to problems with the dialysis solution. These include: overheating, hypotonicity due to an insufficient concentrate-to-water ratio, contamination with formaldehyde, bleach, chloramine, or nitrates from the water supply, and copper from copper tubing or piping. Red blood cell trauma due to improperly functioning roller clamps on dialysis machines, kinking of the blood lines, and poorly constructed blood tubing can also occur.

Hemolysis may also be caused by bypassing arterial pillows, which are still utilized to monitor for excessive pressure in some dialysis units. The initial treatment of suspected hemolysis in a patient on hemodialysis is to stop dialysis immediately, clamp the blood lines (do not return the blood to avoid increasing the risk of hyperkalemia), prepare to treat hyperkalemia and the potentially severe anemia, and investigate the cause. Patients require hospitalization for observation since life-threatening hyperkalemia may develop after dialysis has been terminated.

Air embolism during hemodialysis is another cause of chest pain as well as other symptoms, particularly dyspnea. It can lead to death unless quickly detected and treated. Fortunately, air embolism is rare in hemodialysis patients, in part because of the presence of air detectors in hemodialysis machines. Foam in the venous blood line should make one suspect that air is entering the dialysis system.

Disconnection of connecting caps and/or blood lines can also lead to air embolism in patients being dialyzed with central venous catheters. Symptoms due to an air embolism depend in part upon the patient's physical position at the time of the event. In the seated patient, air tends to migrate into the cerebral venous system without entering the heart; in those who are recumbent, air tends to first enter the heart and then the lungs.

As a result, the seated patient with an air embolism may lose consciousness and seize, while the recumbent patient may initially develop dyspnea, cough, and perhaps chest tightness. Subsequent acute neurologic and cardiac dysfunction in the recumbent patient may be due to the direct passage of air into the arterial system, paradoxical embolization, or incomplete filtering of a large air embolus by the pulmonary capillaries. Treatment of suspected air embolism includes clamping the venous line and stopping the blood pump. The patient should be positioned on the left side in a supine position with the chest and head tilted downward.

Cardiorespiratory support, the administration of 100 percent oxygen by either mask or endotracheal tube, and attempted percutaneous aspiration of air from the ventricle may be required. The most important aspect of air embolism is prevention; this is accomplished through the adequate function of monitoring devices on dialysis machines.

Arrhythmias

The occurrence of ventricular arrhythmias in dialysis patients has been evaluated by Holter monitoring. These arrhythmias are common during dialysis and between treatments; the published frequency ranges widely from 5 to 75 percent. Supraventricular arrhythmias are also common. Risk factors for arrhythmias and sudden death in dialysis patients include coronary artery disease, advanced age, myocardial dysfunction, and left ventricular hypertrophy.

Patients with underlying autonomic dysfunction are also at greater risk of arrhythmias. A higher prevalence of conduction defects, particularly first degree atrioventricular block and bundle branch block, has been associated with mitral valve or mitral annular calcification. During hemodialysis, the incidence of arrhythmias may be enhanced because of rapid fluctuations in hemodynamics and electrolyte concentrations, as well as the induction of hypoxemia in patients with a high incidence of myocardial disease. Studies examining the role of potassium in dialysis-induced arrhythmias are somewhat contradictory, but new techniques may lead to a better understanding of the interactions of potassium, hemodialysis, and arrhythmias. Some reports have found no relationship of plasma potassium to the development of arrhythmias, and the use of low potassium dialysate has been reported to be safe. The treatment of arrhythmias that occur in hemodialysis patients, either during or between hemodialysis sessions, is similar to their treatment in the nondialysis patient. However, appropriate dosing of medications based upon the absence of renal function is always required.

Dyspnea

Patients may complain of shortness of breath while on hemodialysis. Most often, the dyspnea will occur as a result of volume overload and the patient will describe the dyspnea as occurring before the start of the hemodialysis treatment. However, dyspnea that begins after the initiation of hemodialysis should prompt consideration of other possible causes such as acute coronary syndrome, bacteremia (associated with dialysis catheter), a reaction to the hemodialyzer, pericardial effusion with or without tamponade, or pneumonia. The presence of simultaneous symptoms (eg, fever, chills, hypotension, cough) often leads to the identification of the cause of the dyspnea.

The timing of onset of dyspnea may also provide clues to its etiology. As an example, pulmonary embolism should be considered if dyspnea occurs after access declotting. Recurrent episodes of dyspnea occurring on dialysis are most likely to be associated with dialyzer reactions or, possibly, heparin-associated effects.

References

Brenner and Rector´s. The Kidney. 8th Edition.Philadelphia: Saunders Elsevier, 2008.

Daugirdas JT, Blake PG, Ing TS. Handbook of Dialysis. 4th Edition. Philadelphia: Lippincott Williams and Wilkins, 2007.

Floege J, Johnson RJ,Feehally J. Comprehensive Clinical Nephrology, 4th Edition. Philadelphia:Mosby Elsevier, 2011.

www.uptodate.com

In: Hemodialysis: Indications, Procedures and Complications ISBN: 978-1-62081-301-0
Editors: Y F. Cabral and M. Costa De Santos

Chapter IV

Prevention of Hemodialysis Catheter-Related Infections

Igor Denizarde Bacelar Marques, Rosilene Motta Elias and Hugo Abensur
Nephrology Division, Department of Internal Medicine,
University of Sao Paulo School of Medicine, Brazil

Abstract

Despite all efforts to reduce the use of catheters in hemodialysis patients because of related complications, the frequency of catheter use continues to rise. Almost 30% of chronic hemodialysis patients are dependent on central venous catheters (CVC) for their vascular access. CVC have significantly higher rates of infection when compared to grafts and fistulae. It has been estimated that the relative risk for infection in tunneled catheters, cuffed, and uncuffed, when compared with native arteriovenous fistulae is 15.5 and 22.5, respectively. Ideally, dialysis centers should have a catheter-related bacteremia rate of less than 1 per 1000 catheter-days. The most important risk factors for catheter-related infections (CRI) include the presence of diabetes, peripheral atherosclerosis, a previous history of bacteremia, nasal carriage of *Staphylococcus aureus*, longer duration of catheter use, and local infection. CRI is an important source of morbidity and mortality in hemodialysis patients, being responsible for the deaths of approximately 2000 to 5000 hemodialysis patients each year in the United States. A recent clinical trial addressing the prevention of CRI demonstrated that 12% of bacteremia episodes resulted in death. The costs to the health care system are also substantial. Data from the United States Renal Data System and Medicare estimated the total costs of CRI may approach 1 billion dollars per year. Several techniques have been used to decrease the incidence of CRI. These include the use of systemic antibiotics around the time of catheter placement, antimicrobial lock solutions, antimicrobial impregnated catheters, exit-site antimicrobials, and agents used to reduce nasal colonization. The main health risks associated with antimicrobial interventions include side effects such as ototoxicity with gentamicin, hypocalcaemia with citrate, and possible emergence of resistant organisms. These interventions also entail additional costs to the health care provider. This review describes the epidemic problem of CRI, and reviews recent clinical trials of antimicrobial interventions for the prevention of CRI and the importance of strict infection prophylaxis protocol based on universal precautions against infection.

Prevention of Hemodialysis Catheter-Related Infections

The arteriovenous fistulae (AVF) is the vascular access of choice for hemodialysis because of its longevity and lower complication rates compared with arteriovenous grafts (AVG) and catheters. However, with the changing demographics of the end-stage renal disease (ESRD) population worldwide, the construction of an adequate AVF in all patients has proven difficult. It has been estimated that almost 30% of chronic hemodialysis patients are dependent on central venous catheters (CVC) for their vascular access [1].

Data from the Dialysis Outcomes and Practice Patterns Study (DOPPS) have shown large international variations in vascular access practice. Greater mortality risks have been seen for hemodialysis (HD) patients dialyzing with a catheter or graft versus a native AVF, after adjusting for demographics, comorbid conditions and laboratory values [2]. A 1.5- to threefold increase in all-cause and infectious mortality with catheter use in the first 6 months of treatment was observed by Polkinghorne and collaborators [3]. In the CHOICE study, incident hemodialysis patients who were using a venous catheter were at a 47% higher risk for death compared with their counterparts who were using an AVF. Patients who were using an AVG were at intermediate risk. This association remained after adjustment for potential confounding factors and after accounting for frequent changes in access type over time [4].

Infectious complications associated with catheter use in hemodialysis patients contributes to infection becoming the second leading cause of death in patients with chronic kidney disease (CKD) [5]. CVC have significantly higher rates of infection when compared to grafts and fistulae. It has been estimated that the relative risk for infection in tunneled catheters (TCC), cuffed and uncuffed, when compared with native AVF is 15.5 and 22.5, respectively [6]. CVC are responsible for almost half of all infections in HD patients even though they represent the smallest fraction of accesses [7]. Rates of mortality from infection in the first year of HD are now 2.4 times greater than in 1981 and this is largely attributed to CVC use. Hospitalizations due to vascular access infections more than doubled between 1993 and 2005 in the United States and mirror the marked increase of CVC use during the same period, suggesting that increased hospitalization may not be solely attributable to poor CVC care but due to increased CVC use itself [8].

The most important risk factors for catheter-related infections (CRI) include the presence of diabetes, peripheral atherosclerosis, a previous history of bacteremia, poor patient hygiene, recent hospitalization, thrombosis, nasal and skin carriage of *Staphylococcus aureus*, longer duration of catheter use, inadequate dialysis, hypoalbuminemia, local infection, iron overload, immune-incompetency, and the conditions of catheter placement [8].

CRI is an important source of morbidity and mortality in hemodialysis patients, being responsible for deaths of approximately 2000 to 5000 hemodialysis patients each year in the United States [9]. A recent clinical trial addressing the prevention of CRI demonstrated that 12% of bacteremia episodes resulted in death [10]. In the WAVE 2 study, a randomly selected prospective cohort of incident dialysis patients was studied to determine whether there was an association between bacteremia or sepsis episodes and subsequent cardiovascular events [11]. They found that these infectious problems were associated with subsequent death (hazards ratio [HR] 2.33, 95% confidence interval [CI] 1.38–2.28), myocardial infarction (HR 1.78, 95% CI 1.38–2.28), heart failure (HR 1.64, 95% CI 1.39–1.95), peripheral vascular disease (HR 1.64, 95% CI 1.34–2.0), and stroke (HR 2.04, 95% CI 1.27–3.28).

The costs to the health care system are also substantial. Data from the United States Renal Data System and Medicare estimated the total costs of CRI may approach 1 billion dollars per year [12, 13].

Categories and Diagnosis of CRI

Infection associated with TCC can be classified into three categories: exit-site infection, tunnel infection and catheter-related bacteremia (CRB). The therapeutic approach to each of these is somewhat different [14].

Exit-Site Infection

An exit-site infection is defined as culture-positive inflammation external to the cuff, localized to the exit site, not extending above the cuff. It is characterized by localized redness, crusting, and a variable amount of exudate. If the patient also has systemic symptoms, systemic infection should be suspected and blood cultures should be obtained. If the blood cultures are positive, the case should be classified as a CRB rather than an exit-site infection. This is a localized infection and in most cases should respond when treated with local measures. As the great majority of these are staphylococcal, mupirocin generally works well. Systemic antibiotics are necessary only in more severe cases characterized by worsening of the local signs of inflammation and the appearance of increasing amounts of drainage. Cases that fail to respond quickly to local measures may necessitate exchange with the creation of a new exit site or removal if that is feasible. Patients with exit site infection should be monitored for the development of tunnel infection or systemic symptoms suggesting the appearance of a CRB.

Tunnel Infection

A tunnel infection is defined as culture-positive inflammation within the catheter tunnel internal to the Dacron cuff with a negative blood culture. Involvement of the tunnel below the cuff is commonly seen as part of the exit-site infection. When the tunnel is infected above the cuff, it is a serious problem because the catheter moves back and forth within this portion of the tunnel and there is direct communication with the bloodstream. Appropriate treatment of a tunnel infection, whether it occurs alone or as an accompaniment to CRB, consists of catheter removal along with parenteral antibiotics chosen according to culture results.

Catheter-Related Bacteremia

CRB is defined as bacteremia in a patient with a catheter and no other explanation for the positive blood culture. According to Recommendations of Centers for Disease Control and Prevention (CDC), CRB diagnosis must be based on the following definitions:

- Definite blood stream infection: the same organism from a semiquantitative culture of the catheter tip (>15 colony-forming units per catheter segment) and from a peripheral or catheter blood sample in a symptomatic patient with no other apparent source of infection.
- Probable blood stream infection: defervescence of symptoms after antibiotic therapy with or without removal of catheter, in the setting in which blood cultures confirm infection, but catheter tip does not (or catheter tip does, but blood cultures do not) in a symptomatic patient with no other apparent source of infection.
- Possible blood stream infection: defervescence of symptoms after antibiotic treatment or after removal of catheter in the absence of laboratory confirmation of bloodstream infection in a symptomatic patient with no other apparent source of infection.

The CDC recommends one of two culture techniques for diagnosing CRB: paired quantitative blood cultures, or paired qualitative blood cultures observing a differential time to positivity (DTP). Both require the simultaneous draw of blood from a peripheral vein and from the catheter. A colony count of microbes grown from blood obtained through the catheter hub that is at least 3-fold greater than the colony count from blood obtained from a peripheral vein best defines CRB. Unfortunately, the use of the quantitative culture technique, although the most accurate, is limited because of its complexity, cost, and lack of methods in most hospitals for performing the test. The DTP method monitors for bacterial growth and compares the time to positivity for both the peripheral and the CVC blood samples. A catheter-drawn blood culture that turns positive 2 hours or more before a simultaneously drawn peripheral blood culture confirms the catheter as the source of infection. The cultures should be drawn, if possible, before beginning systemic antibiotics, to avoid false-negative peripheral cultures. However, this seemingly basic requirement has been challenging because of the unique circumstances of HD patients, whereby the rigorous standard of requiring quantitative blood cultures and/or DTP from a peripheral vein and catheter blood culture cannot be obtained because of logistic or other reasons. For example, the priority of preserving arm veins for future fistula creation, fragile and damaged vessels, and patient refusal render venipuncture impractical. The IDSA (Infectious Diseases Society of America) has recently acknowledged these significant challenges, and provision has been made to accept blood cultures obtained from the catheter and blood line connected to the CVC (instead of peripheral vein venipuncture) when peripheral vein samples are not possible. Drainage at the CVC exit site should be cultured as the diagnosis of CRB is strengthened by a positive culture of the same organism at the exit site and in the blood [15].

Incidence of CRB

The true incidence of CRB associated with TCC is not known. A relatively broad range has been reported, undoubtedly related to variations in practice patterns. It is clear, however, that the rate is less than that seen with uncuffed (acute) catheters, but not a great deal lower. Uncuffed catheters have a reported rate of infection ranging from 3.8 to 6.6 episodes / 1000 catheter-days, compared with TCC, with 1.6 – 5.5 episodes / 1000 catheter-days [8, 10, 14, 16]. Rates as low as 1 /1000 catheter-days at risk have been achieved with detailed catheter protocols, demonstrating that it is possible to affect the rate with good clinical practices [17]. Programs with greater rates of infection in long-term catheters should institute continuous quality improvement analysis techniques in order to decrease this incidence. Any program with a rate exceeding 2 /1000 catheter-days has room for improvement (Table 1).

Much of the morbidity and mortality related to catheter infection is due to metastatic infection which has ranged in frequency from 3.2% to 50% in various reports, depending somewhat upon the type of organism involved [14,18]. The risk is higher (41% in one study) with *S. aureus* infection [19]. Such secondary systemic complications as septic arthritis, osteomyelitis, thrombophlebitis, endocarditis, large atrial thrombi, and epidural abscess can occur. Although in most reported series the incidence of these complications is relatively low, they have great gravity because of their severe consequences [8, 14].

Microbiology

Gram-positive organisms are responsible for most CRI. Staphylococcal infection, both coagulase-negative and *S. aureus*, accounts for 40–81% of cases in reported studies [14, 18, 20]. Methicillin-resistant *S. aureus* (MRSA) infection has become increasingly important in these cases. This is underscored by a report based upon data derived from the Active Bacterial Core Surveillance system which indicated that in 2005 the incidence of invasive MRSA infection among dialysis patients was 45.2 cases per 1000 patients. This compares with the general population in which rates of invasive MRSA have ranged from 0.2 to 0.4 infections per 1000 [21].

The remaining infections are due predominantly to enterococci and gram-negative rods. In one study, one-third of the cases of CRB were due to gram-negative rods, with *Enterobacter* and *Pseudomonas* leading the list [22]. Polymicrobial infections may be seen. This was reported in 17% of cases in one study [23].

Table 1. Catheter-related bacteremia rates

< 1 / 1000 catheter-days	Excellent
1 – 2 / 1000 catheter-days	Good
3 – 5 / 1000 catheter-days	Fair
> 6 / 1000 catheter-days	Poor

Adapted from reference 14.

Prevention

There are several opportunities for infection to be introduced in the life of a TCC: catheter placement, open surgical site contamination, exit-site infection, and hub contamination at time of use. Any of these can result in infection and lead to CRB. Infection prophylaxis must be practiced for each.

Skin Antisepsis

Skin antisepsis prior to catheter insertion procedure is critical to infection prophylaxis. Studies have shown that preparation of central venous sites with a 2% aqueous chlorhexidine gluconate lowered CRB rates compared with site preparation with 10% povidone-iodine or 70% alcohol [24, 25]. In 2002 the CDC recommended that 2% chlorhexidine be used for skin antisepsis prior to catheter insertion. The antiseptic should be allowed to remain on the insertion site and to air dry before catheter insertion [26].

Catheter Placement Procedure

It is essential that all TCC be placed under conditions of maximal sterile barrier precautions. The use of a surgical cap and mask, sterile gown, sterile gloves, and a large sterile drape during the insertion of a TCC substantially reduces the incidence of infection compared with standard precautions with only sterile gloves and small drapes [27]. Problems associated with catheter insertion should be suspected in any case in which CRB occurs within the first 72 hours.

Although the administration of systemic antibiotics at the time of catheter insertion is a common practice in some institutions, studies have demonstrated that oral or parenteral antibacterial or antifungal drugs do not reduce the incidence of CRB [28].

Exit-Site Infection

Migration of skin organisms at the insertion site into the cutaneous catheter tract with colonization of the catheter has been thought to be the most common route of infection for peripherally inserted, short-term catheters. However, with a cuffed catheter, a well healed and incorporated cuff arrests this migration (although colonization may well occur prior to this time) [14].

Contamination of the Catheter Hub

Contamination of the catheter hub at the time of use is felt to be a major factor in the pathogenesis of CRB associated with TCC. This leads to colonization of the inner surfaces of the catheter and the formation of a biofilm. There are several opportunities for this contamination to occur. If the gap between the catheter hub and the cap is not adequately cleansed prior to connecting the blood lines, it can be a source of contamination. Allowing the exposed end of the hub to make contact with a non-sterile surface during the hook-up procedure, or just allowing it to lie exposed to the air for a prolonged period can invite problems. Improper cleansing of the hub, touching it with a non-sterile object (hand), or breathing on it by the patient or nurse can result in an infection [14].

Exposing the catheter hub to the breath of the patient or dialysis facility personnel is a major problem and nasal colonization by staphylococcus is the culprit. The incidence of nasal colonization is 10–20% in the normal population and evidence suggests that it is higher among medical workers, including dialysis personnel [29, 30]. *S. aureus* carriage has received attention in the literature as a possible source of infection in HD patients. A recently published trial looked at the carriage of MRSA and subsequent infection among dialysis patients, healthcare workers and their families within a single dialysis center [31]. The investigators found that 36% of colonized subjects went on to develop MRSA infection with the same molecular phenotype as the colonizing strain. Two trials have reported a decrease in incidence of *S. aureus*-related infections with eradication of *S. aureus* carriage [32, 33]. However, neither of these trials included patients with HD catheters and therefore we currently do not have evidence regarding the effectiveness of eradicating *S. aureus* carriage on the reduction of HD CRI.

Manufacturers' directions should be adhered to for the types of disinfectants recommended for safe cleaning of the skin and device. If not contraindicated, the CDC recommends use of 2% chlorhexidine, shown to be superior to povidone-iodine. Careful attention to hub care can decrease the CRB rate almost 4-fold to a rate approaching 1 episode / 1000 catheter-days [5, 26].

Daily Catheter Care

Care given to the catheter after placement is important. This involves several principles: wound care until the surgical site has healed, site cleansing, and the use of a site bandage. The Centers for Disease Control and Prevention (CDC) has no preference between transparent dressing and gauze, except in the case in which the exit site is oozing, which requires gauze. Standard practice is to clean the exit site and redress at each dialysis treatment. A protocol for accomplishing this task in an optimal manner as described by the National Kidney Foundation Clinical Practice Guidelines and Recommendations on Vascular Access is detailed in the Table 2 [5].

A 2010 Cochrane review evaluated the benefits and harms of prophylactic topical antimicrobials, topical antiseptics, medicated and non-medicated dressings on infectious complications among hemodialysis patients with CVC. The authors' conclusions were that mupirocin ointment appears effective in reducing the risk of catheter-related bacteraemia. Insufficient reporting on mupirocin resistance was noted and that needs to be considered in future studies. A lack of high quality data on the routine use of povidone-iodine ointment, polysporin ointment and topical honey warrant larger RCT. Insufficient data also were available to determine which dressing type (transparent polyurethane or dry gauze dressing) has the lowest risk of catheter-related infections [34].

Table 2. Considerations for accessing catheters and cleansing catheter exit-sites

Prepare procedure site using dialysis precautions.

Conduce procedure using aseptic technique (correct hand-washing, masks for patient and staff, "no touch" technique, and disposable clean gloves.

Clorhexidine 2% with 70% alcohol for cleansing of long-term catheter sites.

For patients with sensitivities to clorhexidine 2% with 70% alcohol, clorhexidine aqueous may be used instead.

For patients with sensitivities to clorhexidine aqueous, povidine solution may be used.

Skin cleansing should include the following steps:

- Apply solution / swab in a circular motion working from the catheter exit-site outwards.
- Cover an area 10 cm in diameter.
- Repeat this step twice. Do not rinse off or blot excess solution from skin.
- Allow solution to dry completely before applying dressing.

To cleanse the connection between any CVC hub and cap use 2 swabs:

- Grasp connection with 1 swab.
- Use second connection to clean from catheter connection up catheter for 10 cm.
- Cleanse hub connection site and cap vigorously with the first swab. Discard swab.
- Do not drop a connection site once it is cleaned.

To cleanse the section of the catheter that lies adjacent to the skin, gently swab the top and undersides of the catheter starting at the exit-site and working outwards.

CVC, central venous catheter.

Antimicrobials Lock Solutions and Exit-Site Antimicrobials

The antimicrobial locking solutions (ALS) have been studied as a prophylactic measure to prevent CRI. The ideal ALS should have the following properties: it should be nontoxic when administered systemically, it should prevent catheter thrombosis, it should be effective against a wide variety of microorganisms, it should be biocompatible with the catheter, it should not lead to antibiotic resistance, and it should be readily available and inexpensive. A variety of solutions have been tried over the last decade, but there is no consensus on the ideal solution [35].

The use of antimicrobial lock solutions (ALS) and exit-site antimicrobials (ESA) significantly reduces the risk and rate of CRB and exit-site infection, and the risk of catheter loss due to any complication. Several meta-analyses have concluded that ALS are effective [17, 28, 36–38]. These studies suggest that the use of ALS reduces the risk of CRB in HD patients by about a factor of 3. With regard to effect of ALS on exit-site infection, the study by Weijmer et al. [10] showed a significant reduction in both the rate and risk for this outcome, whilst others did not. Currently, we do not have sufficient evidence to draw conclusions regarding the effectiveness of antimicrobial coating or impregnation of HD catheters or peri-operative systemic administration of antibiotics in the form of intravenous vancomycin for the reduction of CRI [28].

There were very limited data to compare the relative clinical efficacy of various antimicrobial interventions in head-to-head clinical trials. One multi-arm study that compared gentamicin and minocycline-EDTA ALS did not find any difference between them in their clinical efficacy [39]. Similarly, exit-site application of honey compared to other antimicrobials (mupirocin and povidone-iodine) was found to be of similar efficacy in the prevention of CRI [28].

Although the use of ALS has demonstrated effectiveness at reducing the incidence of CRB, there continues to be a hesitance to their overall use, likely due to the concern for the potential for development of drug resistance. The studies that addressed the use of antimicrobials for the prevention of CRI were of relatively short duration, with most of them lasting < 1 year, and the patient numbers were relatively small. It is therefore not possible to state that the use of ALS in the long term will be risk-free from a drug resistance point of view [28].

ALS containing gentamicin are extremely effective in preventing infection; the high concentrations achievable within the catheter are toxic to staphylococci. ALS containing gentamicin are inexpensive and highly effective. Unfortunately, the use of these solutions has been discouraged because of the potential risk for antimicrobial resistance [35]. Another concern with respect to gentamicin ALS is ototoxicity. Almost 10% of the patients in a study of Dogra et al. [40] experienced ototoxicity; however, the authors used a higher concentration of gentamicin (40 mg/ml). This systemic exposure was not seen in another study performed by McIntyre et al. [41], which used a concentration of 5 mg/ml. This is felt to most likely result from leakage of the locking solution from the catheter. Such leakage has been shown to occur with heparin solutions even when the catheter is under-filled [42]. Dogra et al. noted that although catheters were not over-filled, gentamicin blood levels suggested significant risk for chronic aminoglycoside exposure and associated ototoxicity [40].

Another concept that has been applied is the use of non-antibiotic antimicrobial solutions to prevent catheter infection. The first of these to be considered was a concentrated citrate solution which was shown to have an active antimicrobial activity. The clinical advantages offered by citrate have been confirmed in at least two meta-analyses [17, 38]. Over time, progressively lower concentrations of citrate have been applied (from 46.7% to 4%) with still significantly better results, even in the latter case, than those obtained with heparin locks. Citrate locks possibly provide a fairly wider therapeutic window than other ALS. However, cases of inadvertent systematic administration resulting in severe hypocalcemia and cardiac arrest have been described. About 10% of the patients reported metallic taste as a side effect when higher concentrations were used [9, 35, 43].

Ethanol may be an effective agent, but there are concerns about thrombosis and compatibility with catheter materials [35]. Taurolidine, a substance that has been used in Europe since the 1970s as an antimicrobial lavage treating peritonitis and a variety of types of wounds, has been used as a locking solution along with sodium citrate to provide anticoagulation. This antimicrobial agent has been found to be effective against a broad range of gram-negative and gram-positive bacteria as well as many types of fungi. Taurolidine appears to be effective and safe and does not appear to carry the risk for side effects that have been reported for some ALS [14]. One report indicated that CRB rates were reduced to 0.20

episodes / 1000 catheter-days. An increased requirement for thrombolytic interventions to maintain catheter patency has been reported, however [44, 45].

Recently Campos et al. reported a well performed, prospective, randomized clinical trial demonstrating the benefit of an ALS containing minocycline and EDTA in the prevention of hemodialysis CRB [46]. Minocycline has fewer important clinical applications, and the authors postulate that resistance to minocycline would be less of a clinical problem compared with other antibiotics that have been used in ALS, including gentamicin. This might be a distinct clinical advantage. The rate of catheter-related bacteremia was 4.3 per 1000 catheter-days in the control group receiving heparin dwells and 1.1 per 1000 catheter days in the minocycline – EDTA group ($P = 0.005$). The rate of catheter removal due to dysfunction was 4.6 per 1000 catheter-days for the minocycline – EDTA group and 3.2 per 1000 catheter-days for heparin-filled catheters ($P = 0.31$). Thus, there were fewer infections and the rate of catheter thrombosis appeared similar.

The 2009 Clinical Practice Guidelines concerning catheter-related infections from the Infectious Disease Society of America did not specifically address the issues of prevention of CRB and the use of antimicrobial catheter lock in hemodialysis patients [15]. The recent position statement by the European Renal Best Practice (ERBP) on hemodialysis catheters and The Renal Association (UK) recommend preventive use of an antimicrobial catheter lock to reduce the rate of CRB (Table 3).

Table 3. Current guidelines with regard to antimicrobial use for the prevention of HD catheter-related infections

Guideline	Recommendation
National Kidney Foundation Kidney Disease Outcomes Quality Initiative (NKF-KDOQI) [5]	Chlorhexidine solutions to be used as first-line agents for exit-site cleaning, with povidone–iodine as an alternative in those unable to tolerate chlorhexidine. Advocates the adherence to Centers for Disease Control guidelines for the prevention of central venous catheter infections. The CDC guidelines recommend the use of ALS in patients who have recurrent bacteraemia and in whom maximum adherence to sterile technique has been determined.
The Renal Association (UK) [47]	Recommends disinfection with chlorhexidine solutions instead of povidone–iodine, and suggest that an antimicrobial or antibiotic lock solution be used to reduce catheter related bacteraemia and other infections.
European Renal Association (ERA-EDTA) [43]	Recommends strict protocols for handling catheters based on aseptic manipulation and mentions that the regular and pre-emptive use of locking solutions (citrate) with both antithrombotic and/or antiseptic properties is effective in preventing catheter infection.
The Evidence-Based Practice in Infection Control (EPIC) [48]	Recommends the use of alcoholic chlorhexidine solution for skin cleansing prior to insertion of central venous catheters and also during handling of such catheters. The EPIC guidelines advocate against the use of ALS and ESA.

While antimicrobials in the form of ALS and exit-site applications have been impressively effective in the reductions of CRI, one should be mindful of addressing basic aspects effectively such as the use of masks and sterile gloves and the use of non-touch techniques. One study has shown that the adoption of a strict aseptic protocol alone significantly reduced the incidence of CRB [49].

Based upon a meta-analysis of prospective randomized trials of ALS used in the prevention of CRB in HD patients, Labriola et al. concluded that the achieved absolute incidence obtained with these solutions was similar to the best-published figures related to careful catheter-use management practices [17]. The NKF-KDOQI guidelines recommend following the CDC guidelines with respect to aseptic handling of catheters, and the EPIC guidelines in the UK make similar recommendations [5, 26, 48].

Aspirin

In vitro studies have shown that salicylic acid, the major metabolite of aspirin, decreases the adherence of staphylococcus to synthetic graft material as well as endothelial cells. Additionally, production of the cytokine, interleukin-6, by endothelial cells appears to be decreased in vitro using salicylic acid [50]. In vivo, aspirin has been shown to cause a reduction in the virulence of *S. aureus*-associated experimental endocarditis [51]. Additionally, studies have shown that the prevalence of nasal carriage of *S. aureus* is significantly lower among patients who receive acetylsalicylic acid when compared with aspirin-free control subjects [52].

Because of these studies, a retrospective analysis of dialysis patients was performed to determine whether the use of aspirin might decrease the frequency of *S. aureus* bacteremia in these cases [53]. The data generated from this analysis revealed that there was a lower rate of catheter-associated *S. aureus* bacteremia in patients treated with aspirin versus those not treated, and this association was dose dependent, being seen mostly with the 325 mg aspirin dose. Additionally, the risk of developing a first episode of *S. aureus* bacteremia was decreased by 54% in patients taking aspirin. Aspirin was also associated with a decreased risk of a first episode of MRSA bacteremia and metastatic complications during the first episode of catheter-related *S. aureus* bacteremia. These results look very promising and need to be confirmed with a prospective randomized clinical trial.

Conclusion

The first logical step of a preventative strategy is to intensify the education of all dialysis unit staff members on adequate daily catheter care. The use of additional prevention methods like ALS could be reserved to patients at high risk of infection (such as diabetics, carriers of femoral catheters or individuals with a history of recurrent CRB), subjects in whom a CRB would lead to dramatic consequences (such as patients with artificial heart valves, pacemakers, vascular grafts, ...), or to units where the rate of CRB has not decreased despite optimal maximal adherence to aseptic technique.

We feel that the judicious use of antimicrobials, especially in the form of ALS and ESA, along with scrupulous attention to aseptic techniques during the handling of HD catheters, can lead to significant reductions in CRI and consequently reduce patient morbidity and mortality, and also reduce the financial burden incurred by the health care providers on account of such infections. However, we need to continue to be vigilant about emergence of a drug-resistant organism and continue to evaluate alternative antimicrobials agents (non-antibiotics) against which resistance is not possible or is clinically irrelevant (e.g. calcium chelators, minocycline-EDTA). Further, adequately powered and well-designed studies assessing the effectiveness of antimicrobial-coated catheters, peri-operative systemic antibiotic usage and a head-to-head trial of various antimicrobials are recommended to inform us regarding their relative effectiveness.

References

[1] Pisoni RL, Young EW, Dysktra DM et al. Vascular access use in Europe and the United States: results from the DOPPS. *Kidney Int.* 2002; 61: 305–316.

[2] Pisoni RL, Arrington CJ, Albert JM et al. Facility hemodialysis vascular access use and mortality in countries participating in DOPPS: an instrumental variable analysis. *Am. J. Kidney Dis.* 2009; 53: 475–491.

[3] Polkinghorne KR, McDonald SP, Atkins RC, Kerr PG. Vascular access and all-cause mortality: A propensity score analysis. *J. Am. Soc. Nephrol.* 2004; 15: 477–486.

[4] Astor BC, Eustace JA, Powe MR, Klage NJ, Fink NE, Coresh J. Type of vascular access and survival among incident hemodialysis patients: the Choices for Healthy Outcomes in Caring for ESRD (CHOICE) Study. *J. Am. Soc. Nephrol.* 2005; 16: 1449–1455.

[5] Vascular Access Work Group. Clinical practice guidelines for vascular access. *Am. J. Kidney Dis.* 2006; 48 (Suppl 1): S248–S273.

[6] Taylor G, Gravel D, Johnston L et al. Prospective surveillance for primary bloodstream infections occurring in Canadian hemodialysis units. *Infect. Control. Hosp. Epidemiol.* 2002; 23: 716–720.

[7] Dittmer ID, Sharp D, McNulty CAM et al. A prospective study of central venous haemodialysis catheter colonization and peripheral bacteraemia. *Clin. Nephrol.* 1999; 51: 34–39.

[8] Lok CE, Mokrzycki MH. Prevention and management of catheter-related infection in hemodialysis patients. *Kidney Int.* 2011; 79: 587–598.

[9] Bleyer AJ. Use of antimicrobial catheter lock solutions to prevent catheter-related bacteraemia. *Clin. J. Am. Soc. Nephrol.* 2007; 2: 1073– 1078.

[10] Weijmer MC, van den Dorpel MA, Van de Ven PJ et al. Randomized, clinical trial comparison of trisodium citrate 30% and heparin as catheter-locking solution in hemodialysis patients. *J. Am. Soc. Nephrol.* 2005; 16: 2769–2777.

[11] Ishani A, Collins AJ, Herzog CA, Foley RN. Septicemia, access and cardiovascular disease in dialysis patients: the USRDS Wave 2 study. *Kidney Int.* 2005; 68: 311–318.

[12] Engemann JJ, Friedman JY, Reed SD et al. Clinical outcomes and costs due to Staphylococcus aureus bacteraemia among patients receiving long-term haemodialysis. *Infect. Control Hosp. Epidemiol.* 2005; 26: 534–539.

[13] Manierski C, Besarab A. Antimicrobial locks: putting the lock on catheter infections. *Adv. Chronic Kidney Dis.* 2006; 13: 245–258.

[14] Beathard GA, Urbanes A. Infection Associated with Tunneled Hemodialysis Catheters. *Semin. Dial.* 2008; 21: 528 – 538.

[15] Mermel LA, Allon M, Bouza E et al. Clinical practice guidelines for the diagnosis and management of intravascular catheter-related infection: 2009 Update by the Infectious Diseases Society of America. *Clin. Infect. Dis.* 2009; 49: 1–45.

[16] Tanriover B, Carlton D, Saddekni S et al. Bacteremia associated with tunneled dialysis catheters: comparison of two treatment strategies. *Kidney Int.* 2000; 57: 2151–2155.

[17] Labriola L, Crott R, Jadoul M. Preventing haemodialysis catheter-related bacteraemia with an antimicrobial lock solution: A meta-analysis of prospective randomized trials. *Nephrol. Dial. Transplant.* 2008; 23: 1666–1672.

[18] Krishnasami Z, Carlton D, Bimbo L et al. Management of hemodialysis catheter-related bacteremia with an adjunctive antibiotic lock solution. *Kidney Int.* 2002; 61: 1136–1142.

[19] Marr KA, Sexton DJ, Conlon PJ, Corey GR, Schwab SJ, Kirkland KB. Catheter-related bacteremia and outcome of attempted catheter salvage in patients undergoing hemodialysis. *Ann. Intern. Med.* 1997; 127: 275–280.

[20] Lok CE, Stanley KE, Hux JE et al. Hemodialysis infection prevention with polysporin ointment. *J. Am. Soc. Nephrol.* 2003; 14: 169–179.

[21] Centers for Disease Control and Prevention (CDC). Invasive methicillin-resistant Staphylococcus aureus infections among dialysis patients – United States. *MMWR Morb. Mortal Wkly. Rep.* 2007; 56: 197–199.

[22] Kovalik EC, Raymond JR, Albers FJ et al. A clustering of epidural abscesses in chronic hemodialysis patients: risks of salvaging access catheters in cases of infection. *J. Am. Soc. Nephrol.* 1996; 7: 2264–2267.

[23] Beathard GA. Management of bacteremia associated with tunneled cuffed hemodialysis catheters. *J. Am. Soc. Nephrol.* 1999; 10: 1045–1049.

[24] Maki DG, Ringer M, Alvarado CJ. Prospective randomized trial of povidone-iodine, alcohol, and chlorhexidine for prevention of infection associated with central venous and arterial catheters. *Lancet* 1991; 338: 339–343.

[25] Chalyakunapruk N, Veenstra DL, Lipsky BA, Saint S. Chlorhexidene compound compared with povidone–iodine solution for vascular catheter site care: a meta-analysis. *Ann. Intern. Med.* 2002; 136: 792–801.

[26] O'Grady NP, Alexander M, Dellinger EP et al. Guidelines for the prevention of intravascular catheter-related infections. *Clin. Infect. Dis.* 2002; 35: 1281–1307.

[27] Raad II, Hohn DC, Gilbreath BJ et al. Prevention of central venous catheter-related infections by using maximal sterile barrier precautions during insertion. *Infect. Control Hosp. Epidemiol.* 1994; 15: 231–238.

[28] Rabindranath KS, Bansal T, Adams J et al. Systematic review of antimicrobials for the prevention of haemodialysis catheter-related infections. *Nephrol. Dial. Transplant.* 2009; 24: 3763–3774.

[29] Choi CS, Yin CS, Bakar AA et al. Nasal carriage of Staphylococcus aureus among healthy adults. *J. Microbiol. Immunol. Infect.* 2006; 39: 458–464.

[30] Karabiber N. Staphylococcus aureus nasal carriage in the normal population and hospital laboratory personnel. *Mikrobiyol. Bul.* 1991; 25: 187–191.

[31] Lu PL, Tsai JC, Chiu YW et al. Methicillin-resistant Staphylococcus aureus carriage, infection and transmission in dialysis patients, healthcare workers and their family members. *Nephrol. Dial. Transplant.* 2008; 23: 1659–1665.

[32] Yu VL, Goetz A, Wagener M. Staphylococcus aureus carriage and infection in patients on haemodialysis. Efficacy of antibiotic prophylaxis. *N. Engl. J. Med.* 1986; 315: 91–96.

[33] Boelaert JR, De Smedt RA, De Baere YA et al. Nasal mupirocin ointment decreases the incidence of Staphylococcus aureus bacteraemias in haemodialysis patients. *Nephrol. Dial. Transplant.* 1989; 4: 278–281.

[34] McCann M, Moore ZE. Interventions for preventing infectious complications in haemodialysis patients with central venous catheters. *Cochrane Database Syst. Rev.* 2010; 20: CD006894.

[35] Bleyer AJ, Murea M. Antimicrobial catheter locks: searching for the ideal solution. *J. Am. Soc. Nephrol.* 2011; 22: 1781–1782.

[36] James MT, Conley J, Tonelli M, Manns BJ, MacRae J, Hemmelgarn BR: Alberta Kidney Disease Network. Meta-analysis: antibiotics for prophylaxis against hemodialysis catheter-related infections. *Ann. Intern. Med.* 2008; 148: 596–605.

[37] Jaffer Y, Selby NM, Taal MW, Fluck RJ, McIntyre CW. A meta-analysis of hemodialysis catheter locking solutions in the prevention of catheter-related infection. *Am. J. Kidney Dis.* 2008; 51: 233–241.

[38] Yahav D, Rozen-Zvi B, Gafter-Gvili A, et al. Antimicrobial lock solutions for the prevention of infections associated with intravascular catheters in patients undergoing hemodialysis: systematic review and meta-analysis of randomized controlled trials. *Clin. Infect. Dis.* 2008; 47: 83–93.

[39] Nori US, Manoharan A, Yee J et al. Comparison of low-dose gentamicin with minocycline as catheter lock solutions in the prevention of catheter-related bacteraemia. *Am. J. Kidney Dis.* 2006; 48: 596–605.

[40] Dogra GK, Herson H, Hutchison B et al. Prevention of tunneled haemodialysis catheter-related infections using catheter-restricted gentamicin and citrate: a randomized controlled study. *J. Am. Soc. Nephrol.* 2002; 12: 2133–2139.

[41] McIntyre CW, Hulme LJ, Taal M et al. Locking of tunneled haemodialysis catheters with gentamicin and heparin. *Kidney Int.* 2004; 66: 801–805.

[42] Sungur M, Eryuksel E, Yavas S, Bihorac A, Layon AJ, Caruso L. Exit of catheter lock solutions from double lumen acute haemodialysis catheters–an in vitro study. *Nephrol. Dial. Transplant.* 2007; 22: 3533–3537.

[43] Vanholder R, Canaud B, Fluck R et al. Diagnosis, prevention and treatment of haemodialysis catheter-related bloodstream infections (CRBSI): A position statement of European Renal Best Practice (ERBP). *NDT Plus* 2010; 3: 234–246.

[44] Quarello F, Forneris G. Prevention of hemodialysis catheter-related bloodstream infection using an antimicrobial lock. *Blood Purif.* 2002; 20: 87–92.

[45] Allon M. Prophylaxis against dialysis catheter-related bacteremia with a novel antimicrobial lock solution. *Clin. Infect. Dis.* 2003; 36: 1539–1544.

[46] Campos RP, Mazza do Nascimento M, Chula DC, Riella MC. Minocycline- EDTA lock solution prevents catheter-related bacteremia in hemodialysis. *J. Am. Soc. Nephrol.* 2011; 22: 1939–1945.

[47] The Renal Association (UK). Clinical guidelines. Vascular Access for Haemodialysis. 2011. Guideline 5.1–5.4. Available at: http://www.renal.org/Clinical/GuidelinesSection/VascularAccess.aspx#Rationale5 (Accessed on 21 December 2011).

[48] Pratt RJ, Pellowe CM, Wilson JA et al. EPIC 2: national evidence based guidelines for preventing healthcare-associated infections in NHS hospitals in England. *J. Hosp. Infect.* 2007; 65S: S1–S64.

[49] Beathard GA. Catheter management protocol for catheter-related bacteraemia prophylaxis. *Semin. Dial.* 2003; 16: 403–405.

[50] Demirag MK, Esen S, Zivalioglu M, Leblebicioglu H, Keceligil HT. The effect of aspirin on adherence of slime-producing, coagulase negative staphylococci to vascular grafts. *Ann. Vasc. Surg.* 2007 21: 464–467.

[51] Kupferwasser LI, Yeaman MR, Nast CC et al. Salicylic acid attenuates virulence in endovascular infections by targeting global regulatory pathways in Staphylococcus aureus. *J. Clin. Invest.* 2003; 112: 222–233.

[52] Karabay O, Arinc H, Gunduz H, Tamer A, Ozhan H, Uyan C. A new effect of acetylsalicylic acid? Significantly lower prevalence of nasal carriage of Staphylococcus aureus among patients receiving orally administered acetylsalicylic acid. *Infect. Control. Hosp. Epidemiol.* 2006; 27: 318–319.

[53] Sedlacek M, Gemery JM, Cheung AL, Bayer AS, Remillard BD. Aspirin treatment is associated with a significantly decreased risk of Staphylococcus aureus bacteremia in hemodialysis patients with tunneled catheters. *Am. J. Kidney Dis.* 2007; 49: 401–408.

In: Hemodialysis: Indications, Procedures and Complications ISBN: 978-1-62081-301-0
Editors: Y F. Cabral and M. Costa De Santos

Chapter V

Complications of Hemodialysis

***Suzanne El-Sayegh**, *Chadi Saifan**,**
Suchita Mehta, Pranab Sharma Acharya, Rabih Nasr and Morton Kleiner
Staten Island University Hospital, Staten Island, NY, US

Introduction

More than 530,000 patients develop end stage renal disease every year in the United States, vast majority requiring hemodialysis (HD). This procedure has become much safer now with the improved water treatments, advent of better dialysis equipment and safety protocols followed during dialysis. However, this procedure still has many complications and adverse events associated with it, most of which occur in the acute setting. The most common complication is hypotension.

Hemodialysis is the most used method of renal replacement therapies. It consists of using the extracorporeal blood circulation. It has the ability to correct the metabolic abnormalities and the uremic symptoms while keeping the fluid status well controlled. It is a lifetime commitment. The patient may need 2 sessions per week, 3 sessions per week or may even need daily treatment depending on numerous factors.

Hemodialysis is not a risk free medical procedure. Complications can occur during the hemodialysis or in between the sessions and can be categorized as "acute complications", or it can occur within months or years after starting hemodialysis and can be categorized as "subacute and chronic complications".

The acute complications that occur during hemodialysis are directly related to the hemodynamic instability, fluid status and the clinical condition of the patient. While some events are expected to happen and can be treated appropriately by the medical team, some others are unpredictable and challenging and can lead to serious outcomes.

* Main authors.

The common acute complications that can happen during hemodialysis are muscle cramps, dialysis dysequilibirium syndrome, hypotension secondary to the cardiovascular instability and fluid shift, headache, loss of balance, nausea, vomiting, and post dialysis fatigue.

The serious complications the can occur during hemodialysis and need a prompt interference by the medical team are: allergic reactions to the sterilizing agent, dialysis material, membrane or even to heparin used to avoid thrombotic events, convulsions and seizures, extrasystolic beats and cardiac arrhythmias, air emboli, fevers, septic shocks, hemolysis and blood dyscrasias. The inter-dialysis complications that occur between the dialysis sessions are: malignant hyperkalemia, increased risk of infection, fluid overload, hemorrhagic events, and ischemic colitis.

The subacute and chronic complications are multiple: inefficient dialysis time related to the absence of improvement of uremic symptoms, iron deficiency anemia, pericarditis, vascular access complications of fistulas, grafts and permanent catheters such as steal syndrome, thrombosis, bleeding and infections.

Training, education, experience and research contribute to the opitimization of the hemodialysis process being largely used by millions of patients worldwide. Avoiding complications and assuring safety are key factors in maintaining adequate hemodialysis. The problems encountered during and after hemodialysis are multiple and not fully understood. For instance, the hemodynamic instability is variable according to each patient's clinical condition.

Providing an adequate dialysis and avoiding complications ameliorate the quality of life, lessen the economic burden and decrease the overall mortality and morbidity. Many protocols, guidelines and policies are being implemented to raise the awareness and decrease the complication rate.

A) Hypotension

Intradialytic hypotension occurs in about 20-30% of all treatments [1]. Hypotension can be a result of multiple factors like ultrafiltration rate, dialysate factors, cardiac causes and some miscellaneous causes like air embolism, occult hemorrhage, septicemia, anaphylactic reactions and intradialytic food ingestion. (See chart 1)

1. *Ultrafiltration* - Hypotension occurring due to ultrafiltration is a result of inadequate vascular refilling and compensation. This vascular refilling varies widely between patients, hence the amount of fluid removal during HD is individualized taking into account their interdialytic weight gain (IDWG) and their estimated dry weight. The following factors contribute to hypotension related to ultrafiltration.
   a) Large interdialytic weight gain – High IDWG leads to excess ultrafiltration and hypotension. Patients should be counseled to limit their salt intake, this being more important than fluid restriction [28]. If this is not possible, the treatment time can be extended with slower removal of fluid or performing HD four times per week can also be considered.

b) Overestimation of dry weight – The most accurate methods for estimation of patient's dry weight like bioimpedance devices, inferior vena cava diameter ultrasonography, serum atrial natriuretic factor levels are usually not used as they are not readily available in the clinical setting. It is, most often, estimated clinically by trial and error method based on the IDWG, edema, patient's blood pressure and the ability to tolerate ultrafiltration. Thus, patients usually have an overestimated dry weight. Also, attempts to reach the goal of true dry weight calculated by the more accurate methods, especially for patients with large IDWG, may result in hypotension.

c) Lack of use of ultrafiltration controller (in the older days) - Fluid removal rate would fluctuate and cause hypotension when this device was not used in the older days but now it is routinely present in dialysis machines.

d) Blood-volume control devices with feedback loop - Feedback devices can reduce the incidence of dialysis-induced hypotension while avoiding a positive sodium balance29.

2. *Dialysate Factors* - The temperature and sodium are most commonly implicated dialysate factors for hypotension. There is a controversy as far as the role of calcium concentration is considered.

a) Higher Dialysate Temperature – This leads to vasodilatation to dissipate heat, decrease in vascular resistance and hypotension. Temperature fluctuation of even 1.1°C can cause significant change in the blood pressure [30]. Temperatures as low as 35 °F can be used, if tolerated by the patient, to maintain the blood pressure especially in patients with cardiac motion abnormalities [2].

b) Low sodium levels in the dialysate solution – This causes hypotonic blood when returning from dialyzer and thus intracellular shift of fluid and decrease in blood volume. This is most pronounced in the early part of HD when there is sudden fall in the sodium level. Thus, there is the "sodium modeling" to prevent this from happening where there is higher concentration of sodium in the dialysate in the beginning of the treatment, with a slow decline in dialysate sodium concentration with the progression of hemodialysis. However, the patient may complete HD with a higher sodium level and have increased thirst [3, 4]. "Individualized" dialysis solution sodium may help in reduction of hypotensive episodes as well as intradialytic thirst [34].

c) Low calcium levels in the dialysate solution – This is a very controversial topic. Higher levels like 1.75mM is associated with increased cardiac function in patients with cardiac dysfunction 5, but on the downside, this level of calcium can cause vascular calcification.

d) Use of acetate as a buffer used in the older days – this has been replaced by bicarbonate containing solutions35.

3. *Cardiac Etiology* - Most commonly diastolic dysfunction.

a) Diastolic dysfunction.

b) Ischemia during HD.

c) Arrhythmia – more commonly atrial.

d) Pericardial tamponade.

4. *Miscellaneous Causes.*

a) Anaphylactic reaction to dialyzer causing hypotension.

b) Autonomic neuropathy.
c) Occult hemorrhage.
d) Sepsis.
e) Hemolysis.
f) Air embolism.
g) Intradialytic food ingestion can cause splanchnic vasodilatation and venous pooling in the splanchnic bed and this effect can last up to two hours [31,32,33].

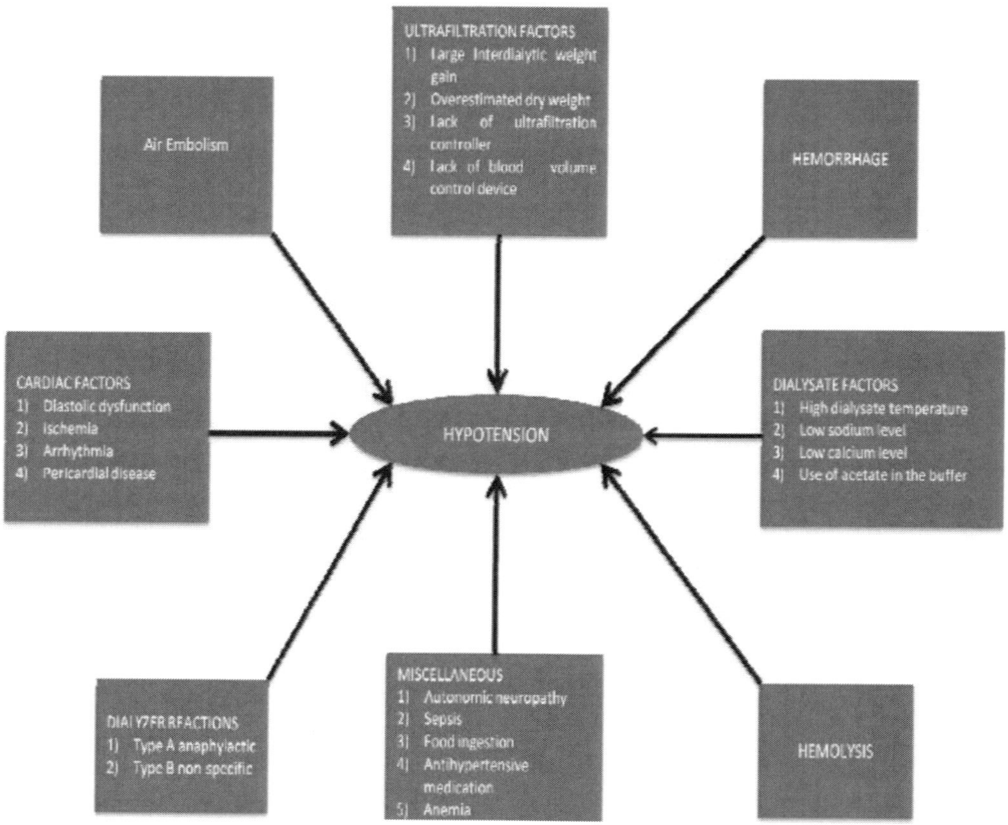

Chart 1. Causes of hypotension.

Management of Hypotension during HD (See Chart 2)

1. *Treatment of an acute episode* - Bolus of 0.9% NS is given, patient is put in Trendelenburg position and the ultrafiltration rate is reduced. The most important step in management of hypotension is to understand the pattern and determine the cause for the individual patient. The next step after having established this is to prevent further episodes in the future by adopting the appropriate strategy.
2. *Prevention of further episodes.*
   a) Limit interdialytic weight gain by counseling the patient to limit salt intake is very important.

b) Reassess dry weight for the patient.
c) Sodium modeling.
d) Use of bicarbonate in the dialysis solution.
e) Use of ultrafiltration controller.
f) Use of blood-volume monitor.
g) Cooler dialysate solution, temperatures as low as 35 -36°F.
h) Avoid food ingestion during dialysis.
i) Administer antihypertensive medications after dialysis.
j) Trial of midodrine.

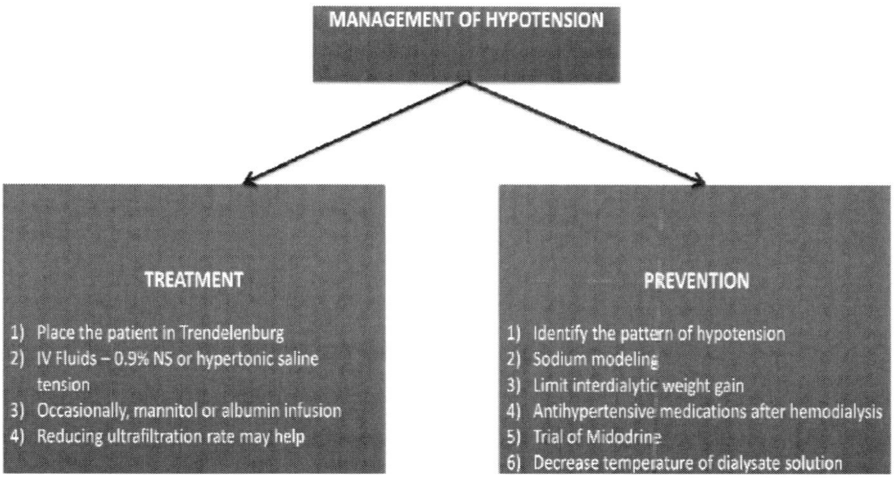

Chart 2. Mmanagement of hypotension.

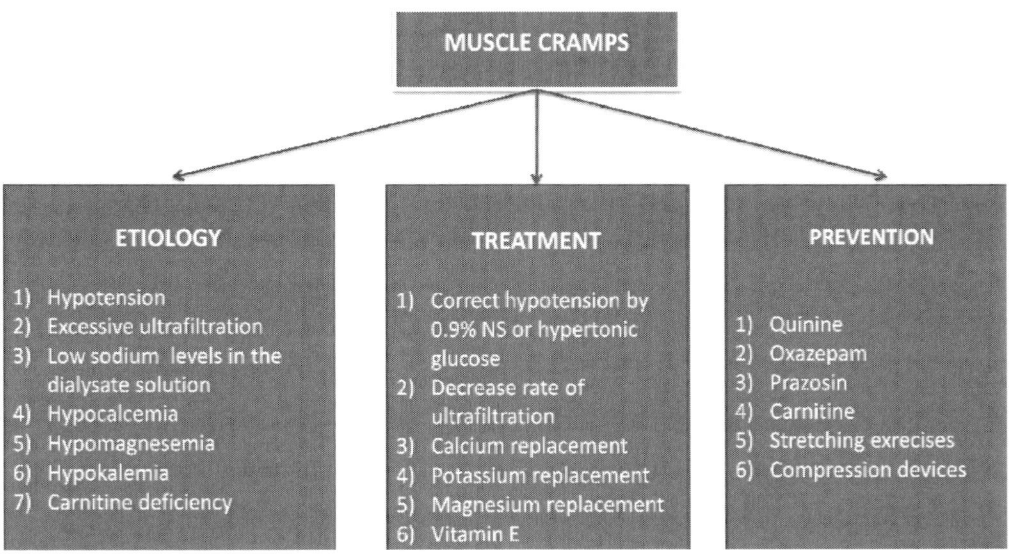

Chart 3. Muscle cramps.

B) Muscle Cramps (See Chart 3)

They occur in 24% to 86% of patients on hemodialysis [36, 37]. The exact pathophysiology of this symptom is not known. It is painful and increases the morbidity. The most common factors are excessive ultrafiltration, hypotension and low sodium concentration in the dialysate solution. Electrolyte abnormalities like hypomagnesemia, hypocalcemia, hypokalemia are also known to produce this symptom. L-carnitine deficiency has been implicated in causing cramps [6] and recently, leptin has also been proposed in the pathophysiology [7].

Treatment of muscle cramps:

1. If hypotension is the reason for the cramps, 0.9% NS can be given even though hypertonic solutions have been shown to be more effective. Hypertonic glucose is the fluid of choice in nondiabetic patients [8].
2. The dry weight for the patient should be reassessed to prevent further episodes of cramps associated with hypotension along with patient education to limit IDWG.
3. Increasing sodium concentration in the dialysate solution to 145 to 155mEq/L and gradual decline to 135 to 140mEq/L or sodium modeling has been shown to beneficial for cramps caused by hyponatremia [12].
4. Quinine has been used frequently to alleviate muscle cramps [9] but due to the side effects it has been removed from over the counter and it is prescribed with black box warning against the use for cramps due its adverse effects. 250 to 325mg of quinine can be given for prevention of cramps.
5. Carnitine supplementation may help (20mg/kg given IV post dialysis or oral carnitine 330mg two or three times per day) [38].
6. Some other medications that can help with cramps are oxazepam, vitamin E [10].
7. Stretching exercise and compression device may provide some relief [11].

C) Dialysis Disequilibrium Syndrome

This syndrome is seen most often seen when acutely uremic patients are dialyzed aggressively. The severe manifestations are not commonly seen now due to improved dialysis strategies. It can manifest with mild symptoms like nausea, vomiting, restlessness and fatigue to severe symptoms like headache, seizures, obtundation or coma. These symptoms usually occur at the end of the treatment but they can present up to 24 hours after HD. The exact mechanism of this syndrome is still unclear.

1. *Pathogenesis.*
   a) Reverse Osmosis - The reasons for this is thought to be due to rapid removal of urea causing drastic fall in plasma osmolality and thus water shifting in the intracerebral cells [13].
   b) Paradoxical intracerebral acidosis - This develops when there is drop in the plasma pH due to dialysis especially made worse when bicarbonate is used [14]. The sudden drastic fall in the osmolality of plasma that occurs with the rapid

removal of urea during dialysis leads to hypotonic plasma in comparison to the brain cells and thereby causing an intracellular fluid shift. Retention of idiogenic osmoles like inositol, glutamine also contributes to this fluid retention within the cells.

2. *Manifestations.*
3. Severe symptoms like seizures, obtundation, coma and death can occur.
4. Milder symptoms like nausea, vomiting, fatigue, headache, restlessness can also due to this syndrome.
5. *Treatment* – The first step in the management for severe manifestations like seizures or change in mental status, is immediate termination of dialysis and administration of mannitol or 5ml of 23% saline to increase the plasma osmolarity. Maintain airway and supportive care is important. These severe symptoms are usually self limiting with the correction of plasma osmolarity and rarely last more than 24 hours.
6. *Prevention* – Disequilibrium can be prevented by slower dialysis for acutely uremic patients with the target reduction in urea being limited to 30%. Higher dialysate sodium concentration decreases the shift of fluid in the brain cells [13]. Other techniques that may help decrease disequilibrium syndrome are use of smaller surface-area dialyzer, low blood flow during the HD, timely initiation of HD for stage V CKD patients, increasing the duration of dialysis by 30 mins.

This entity is self limited in majority of the cases but sometimes patients take several days to recover fully.

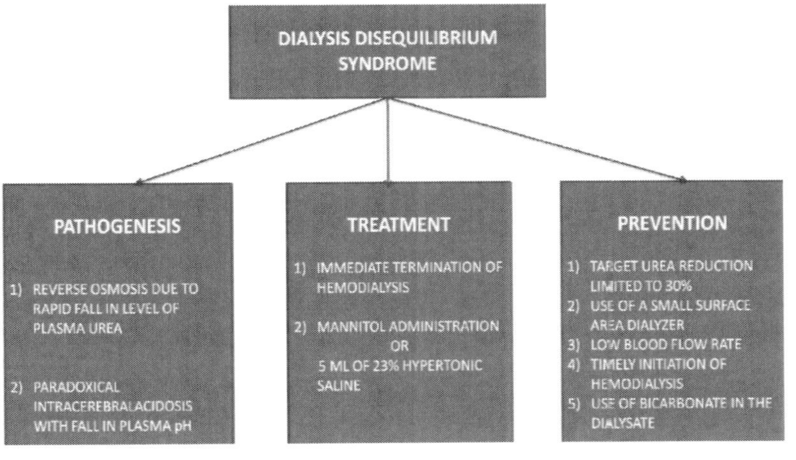

Chart 4. Disequilibrium syndrome.

D) Dialyzer Reactions

Dialyzer reactions in the past were called "first –use reactions" but later it was known that these reactions occur with reused filters. These reactions are classified into two types: Type A (anaphylactic type) and type B (non- specific) [1]. (See chart 7).

1. Type a Reaction

This is an anaphylactic type of reaction mediated by IgE and consists of itching, urticaria, sneezing and watery eyes. Anaphylactic and anaphylactoid reactions usually occur within 5 to 20 minutes. It can sometimes be life-threatening with angioedema, laryngeal edema and respiratory failure. It can also manifest with gastrointestinal symptoms like nausea, vomiting, abdominal pain and diarrhea. The etiology for this reaction is multiple and consists of the following:

a) Ethylene oxide – used as sterilizing agent in the past but now most of the machines are sterilized with agents that have minimal ethylene oxide. Radioallergosorbent test (RAST) test to detect specific IgE antibodies can be use but 10% of patients with no history of dialysis reactions have a positive RAST result39.
b) Reuse reactions – These are mainly due to the disinfectants that are used to clean the reused dialysis instruments. These disinfectants include formaldehyde, glutaraldehyde and peracetic acid-hydrogen peroxide40.
c) AN69 membrane – This is seen particularly in patients receiving ACE inhibitors. The reaction is due to bradykinin which is activated by this negatively charged membrane and levels are further increased due to ACE inhibitors [15, 16, 41].
d) Drug Reactions - Allergic reaction to heparin can cause an anaphylactoid reaction and heparin-free dialysis or citrate anticoagulation should be considered [1]. An outbreak of dialyzer reactions in the USA a few years back was thought to be due contaminated heparin (oversulfated with chondroitin sulfate) 42.
e) Eosiniphilia – Patients with eosinophilia are more prone to type A reactions

Managing these reactions consists of immediate discontinuation of HD, clamping of the lines, no blood return to the patient and cardiopulmonary support, epinephrine, use of corticosteroids. Preventing further reactions is done by identifying the culprit of the reaction and preadministration of antihistamines may be beneficial.

2) Type B Reactions

It is a nonspecific reaction that results due to complement activation and typically presents with chest pain, back pain within 20 to 40 minutes of initiation of the treatment [17]. This reaction is known to occur due to complement activation due to the exposure of the hydroxyl groups on the cellulose membranes. The complement fragments cause migration of neutrophils to lung tissue. There may be transient neutropenia as a result of this and the counts usually increase 30 to 60 minutes after dialysis. This complement activation can be the cause of chest pain, back pain and nausea in patients with a reaction to the cellulose membranes. But nowadays, synthetic membranes like polysulfone, polycarbonate, and polymethylmethacrylate are used and these do not cause such a reaction because the hydroxyl group is covered [43]. Underlying myocardial ischemia should be ruled out. Use of a different membrane might help prevent further episodes. This used to be more prevalent in the earlier days when cellulose membranes were used but now with polyacrylonitrile and polysulfone materials, the rates have gone down. (See chart 5).

3) Febrile Reactions Due to Bacterial Contamination

The probable source of fever in a patient should be identified. It can be a result of any of the following:

a) Catheter related infection.
b) Access via infected arteriovenous grafts or fistula for dialysis [44].
c) Contamination of water used for the treatment.
d) Inadequate sterilization of the dialysis instruments.
e) Systemic infection and bacteremia.

Management of febrile reactions [45,46,47]: (see chart 6 below).

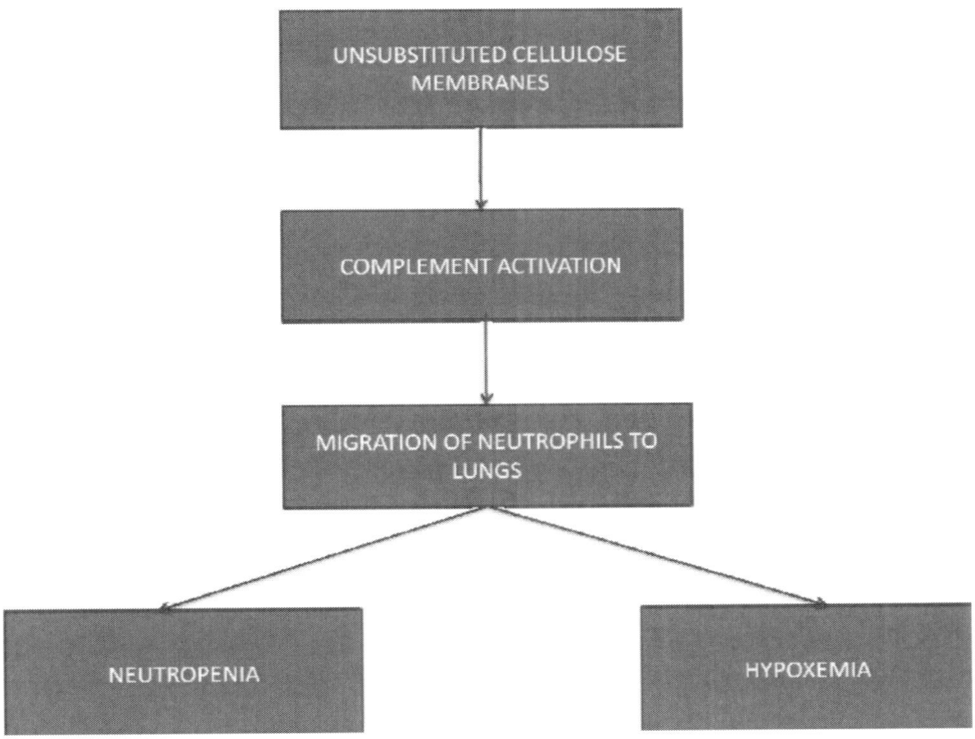

Chart 5. Type b dialyzer reaction.

E) Arrhythmias, Ischemia, Sudden Cardiac Death

1. *Arrhythmias* – The fluctuation in the serum potassium complicated by the use of digoxin plays a major role in the development of arrhythmia, especially when the levels become critically low [18]. Low levels of calcium, magnesium, bicarbonate also contribute to arrhythmia. In addition to these electrolyte disturbances, structural heart disease like uremic pericarditis, left ventricular dysfunction, calcification of the conduction system are also implicated [19, 20].

2. *Sudden Cardiac Death* – This occurs in about seven per 100000 sessions and more common in the elderly and diabetics 21. The most common cause is ventricular arrhythmia however; occasionally it can be due to technical failure like air embolism [22, 23].
3. *Ischemia* – This may present in the absence of typical symptoms and signs [24].

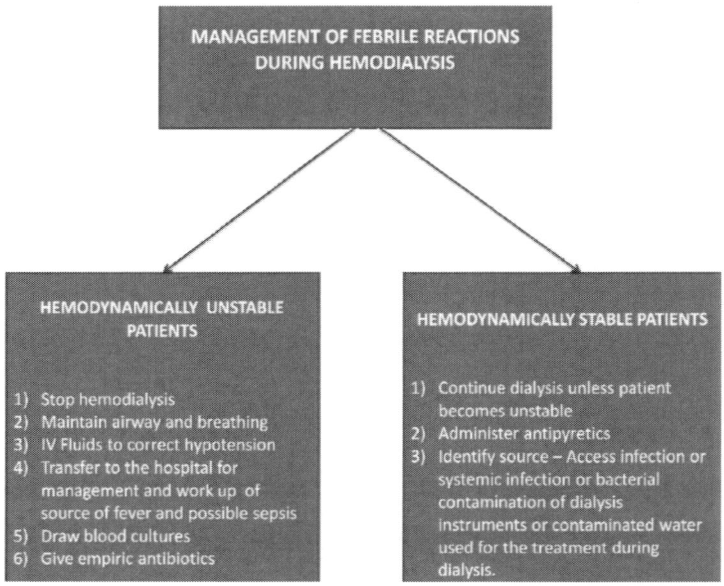

Chart 6. Febrile reactions.

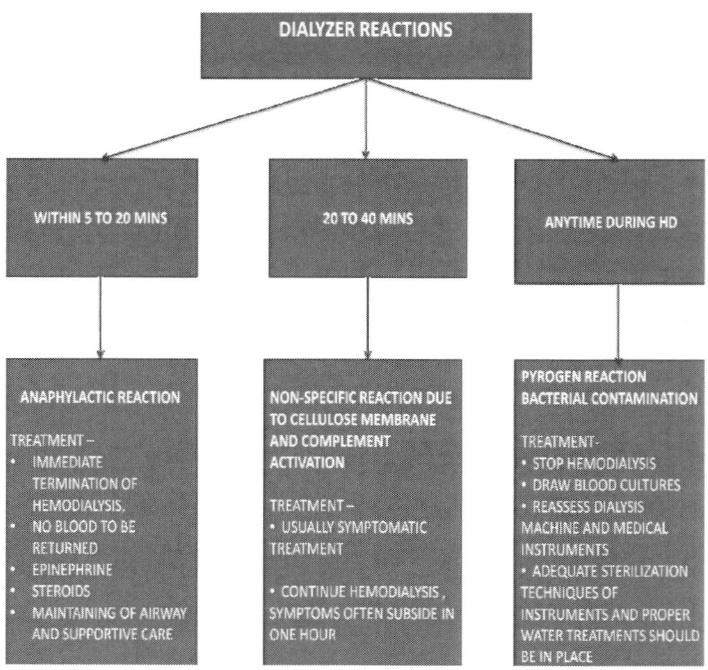

Chart 7. Dialysis reactions.

F) Nausea, Vomiting

It occurs in 10% of treatments and increases the morbidity. The most common cause is hypotension. Some of the other causes include disequilibrium syndrome, dialyzer reactions, dialysis induced worsening of preexisting gastroparesis, narcotics. Patients on hemodialysis experience nausea more readily compared to other patients. It is important to treat hypotension to relieve the nausea. Antiemetics prior to hemodialysis can help preventing nausea that occurs with hemodialysis [1].

G) Headache

It is a common complaint and the exact cause is unclear. Besides disequilibrium syndrome, some frequent causes include caffeine withdrawal and hypomagnesemia. Advising patients to drink coffee during HD, sodium modeling, reducing blood flow rate, repletion of magnesium in deficient patients are some of the measures adopted to decrease further episodes 1.

H) Chest Pain and Back Pain

It occurs in 1% to 4% of treatments. It is important to rule out type B dialyzer reaction and underlying myocardial ischemia when the patient starts complaining of chest and back pain. These symptoms may be present, often, without a clear etiology.1

I) Itching

There are many causes like allergic reaction to dialyzer membrane, new drugs, elevated calcium and phosphorus product. Sometimes, one cannot find the cause and it may be due to dialysis itself. Some of the proposed treatments to relieve itching include gabapentin 25, nalfurafine 26, increased dose of dialysis, use of high flux membrane. Symptomatic relief with antihistamines is important.

J) Seizures [48]

Seizure is not uncommon in dialysis patients. It may be focal or generalized. Intracranial hemorrhage may lead to focal seizures whereas uremic encephalopathy and severe disequilibrium syndrome causes generalized seizures. Metabolic causes include aluminum encephalopathy, hypocalcemia, hypernatremia, air embolism and severe hypotension. Other causes may include dialytic removal of anticonvulsant drugs as well as the use of erythropoesis stimulating drugs. (see chart 8).

Prevention of seizures can be done by measuring predialysis BUN and electrolytes level. Rapid correction of electrolyte abnormality and limiting initial dialysis sessions length and blood flow rate are other approaches to prevent seizures in susceptible patients.

Management: The initial management includes stopping the dialysis. After securing the airway, breathing and circulatory status it is important to measure the electrolytes level. Intravenous glucose should be given if hypoglycemia is suspected. Intractable seizure requires anti-epileptics (diazepam or phenytion). If phenytion is to be started, constant telemetry monitoring should be done to identify potential cardiovascular arrhythmia caused by phenytion.

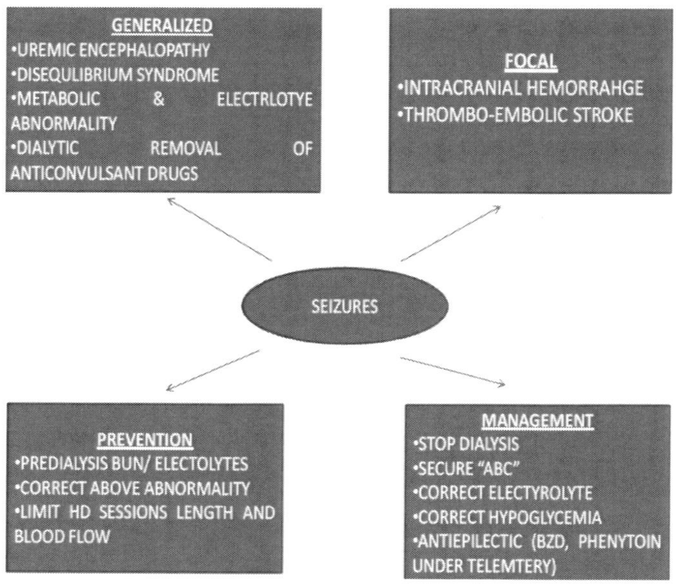

Chart 8. Seizures.

K) Restless Legs Syndrome (RLS)

Restless leg syndrome is common among dialysis patients, with a reported prevalence of 6-60% (SM., 2011). RLS is a subjective feeling described as an irritating sensation deep in the muscles of the lower leg (mainly the calf muscle). It is relieved by moving the lower extremity. Hyperphosphatemia, anxiety, and emotion-oriented coping with stress are related to the presence of RLS during HD. (Takaki J, 2003). Diagnosis is based on brief interview with the patient and their bed partners. Sleep studies (polysomnography) also contribute. (see chart 9).

Management: Iron supplements, regular physical work out, massage are ancillary approaches. L-Dopa and benzodiazepines are other options used.

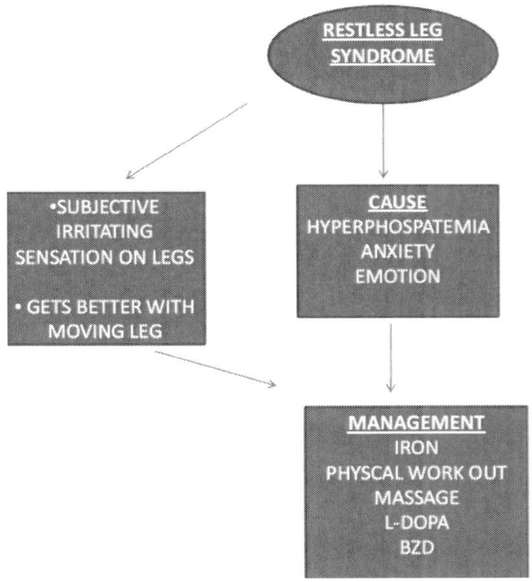

Chart 9. Restless legs syndrome.

L) Uremic Neuropathy

It is one of the chronic complications of HD. Typically it is a distal, symmetric mixed (motor/sensory) polyneuropathy. Clinically it may appear as paresthesia, ataxia and weakness. It is thought to be related to toxin retainment in uremia that is not adequately removed by dialysis. With adequate dialysis this complication is uncommon but if clinical symptoms occur then adequacy of dialysis should be carefully evaluated using kinetic modeling. More frequent dialysis using high-flux membrane or hemodiafiltration increases removal of toxins. (see chart 10).

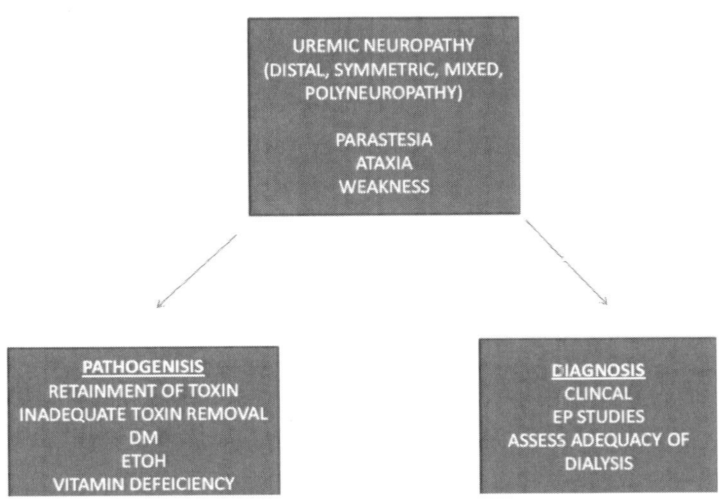

Chart 10. Uremic neuropathy.

Diagnosis: Is usually clinic and Electrophysiology studies (EPS) of motor and sensory nerves aid diagnosis. Other causes of similar symptoms should be considered including DM, alcohol abuse and various vitamin deficiencies.

M) Pruritis

Itching may be an acute or chronic problem in patients with dialysis. Numerous causes have been implicated. It may be a hypersensitivity reaction to dialyzer, hemocircuit components or a manifestation of high PTH with high calcium- phosphorous product.

Management: Reduction in levels of phosphorus, calcium or PTH is indicated where the levels are high. Symptomatic relief can be obtained with anti-histaminics, local emollients, ultraviolet light treatment (JD, DM, A, 3rd, and JP., 1985) and even accupunture. Though many other ancillary treatments are tried, including increasing frequency of sessions, polymethylmethacrylate (PMMA) membrane, erythropoietin- their efficacy remains controversial. Gabapentin use has shown some benefits in recent studies (AI, G, TK, SY, E, and H., 2004).

N) Air Embolism

Air embolism during dialysis has a high mortality rate (Manuel MA, 1972). The pre-tubing segment is where significant subatmospheric pressure exists. This part is most vulnerable to air entry in the extracorporeal segment circuit as air gets sucked into the tubing. Others source of air embolism include bubbles in the dialysate and catheter.

The volume and speed of air introduced in addition to the site where air has been introduced contributes to the symptomatology of air embolism. Large amount of air introduce into the venous circulation is not miscible in blood and travels against gravity. In the sitting position, air entered into the veins can bypass the heart and cause cerebral hypo-perfusion. Seizures and even coma can ensue. This should be suspected in someone who has symptoms of cerebral hypo perfusion with no chest pain or shortness of breath. If the patient is in supine position, the air embolus may not rise to the brain but rather enter the right side of the heart causing obstruction and cardiogenic shock. More disseminated micro-emboli leads to shortness of breath, cough, chest pain complicated with severe hypoxia leading to acute respiratory failure. If the patient is in Trendelunburg position, the air embolus may travel to the lower extremity getting embedded in the venous side. This leads to an increased forward resistance causing obstruction of forward flow and culminating in limb ischemia.

Prevention: The dialyzer machine is equipped with air bubble traps and foam detectors. A venous monitor is used to monitor pressure at the venous end. The dialyzer system is usually attached with an air detector that alarms and closes down the pump after clamping the venous line if air is detected. It is important to withhold any dialysis if alarm was set up. To remove any possible air bubbles, it is important to flush tubing with saline and rinse carefully before connecting patient.

Management: The symptoms of air embolism depend on the position of the patient. So it is important to identify the spectrum of symptoms earlier on. If symptoms suggest air embolism, the venous side has to be clamped as soon as possible and blood pump be stopped. The patient then needs to be placed on a left sided Trendelenburg position to sequester air in the right ventricle. This allows some time for the air to be reabsorbed. Cardiopulmonary support should be given with oxygen and ventilator support as required. A percutaneous needle aspiration of air from the right ventricle could also be attempted. A right atrial catheter can also be used for the same. Hyperbaric oxygenation treatment may be attempted if facilities available.

O) Complication Associated with Urgent Venous Access

Two currently available classes of devices are used for urgent venous access.

- Non- tunneled dialysis catheters.
- Cuffed, tunneled dialysis catheters.

The complication for non- tunneled dialysis catheters may be divided as:

- Insertion complication.
- Catheter thrombosis.
- Central vein thrombosis and stenosis.
- Infection.

Insertion Complication

Lowest rate of complications is at femoral sites and includes perforation and bleeding of the vessel. This can be managed by pressure over the site for 10 to 15 minutes. Hematomas (femoral or retroperitoneal) may also occur if both the walls of vein are penetrated.

Subclavian site insertion has more serious complication. Transient arrhythmia (due to over inserted guidewire), hemothorax, pericardial rupture and tamponade are known complications. Pneumothorax can occur in 1- 10 % of the cases and is greater on the left side than the right (Fan, 1994). Thus, right internal jugular vein is a more preferred. Ultrasound guided insertion minimizes complication risk. (Kwon TH, 1997).

Catheter Thrombosis

Prevention of catheter thrombosis is attempted with instilled heparin following HD. The amount of heparin depends on the length of the catheter and should be just enough to fill the catheter avoiding systemic anticoagualtion. Use of warfarin (Wilkieson TJ, 2011) and tPA (recombinant tissue type plasminogen activator) to prevent thrombosis is under investigation (Macrae JM, 2005). (Hemmelgarn BR and Group., 2011) In established thrombosis, lytic agents (e.g. urokinase (Donati G, 2011) and alteplase are effective. But if flow is inadequate, then non cuffed catheters may need to be replaced.

Central Vein Thrombosis

Central venous canulation creates a nidus of vascular injury leading to fibrosis. The blood flow within the catheter is rapid and creates turbulence leading to endothelial proliferation resulting in venous stenosis (Schwab SJ, 1988). The right internal jugular vein is preferred because of relatively straighter course to subclavian vien.

Management

Thrombolytic therapy or percutaneous transluminal angioplasty with or without stents are the available treatment option once thrombosis is established.

P) Malnutrition

The nutritional status of patients on dialysis is directly related to the incidence of complications, mortality and morbidity. Numerous factors can be involved in the nutritional status of the patients on dialysis including the socioeconomic status, lack of dietary specialists, and depression. It can be assessed and monitored by following blood levels of many makers such as albumin and prealbumin. The nutritional support is crucial because of the multiple medical factors and complications that can result from lack of nutrients. This complication can be well monitored not just by makers, but also by having a nutritionist in every dialysis center to provide counseling.

Q) Gastrointestinal Bleeding

The gastrointestinal complications are frequent in patients on dialysis. Predisposing medical conditions such as prior peptic ulcer disease increase the risk of subsequent complication. Developing gastritis with possible gastrointestinal hemorrhage is a frequent complication in patients on dialysis and should be suspected in every patient having a drop in the hemoglobin level [49]. Some medications such as proton pump inhibitors and anti-H2 receptors can be used to decrease the incidence of these complications. Blood related abnormalities are frequent in patients on dialysis especially hemolysis.

R) Psychiatric Complications

Dialysis requires a continuous treatment for toxins removal. Some patients will have to leave their jobs and be on disability because of these requirements. The change in lifestyle and the adaptation to a different living situation may impose a lot of emotional pressure leading to depression and anxiety. Psychological and psychosocial supports are fundamental in avoiding a subsequent depression.

References

[1] Daugirdas JT, Blake PG and Todd S. *Handbook of dialysis.* 3rd edition. Lippincott Williams and Wilkins, Hagerstown, MD: 2001.

[2] Selby NM, Burton JO, Chesterton LJ, et al. Dialysis-induced regional left ventricular dysfunction is ameliorated by cooling the dialysate. *Clin. J. Am. Soc. Nephrol.* 2006;1:1216-1225.

[3] Song JH, Park GH, Lee SY, et al. Effect of sodium balance and the combination of ultrafiltration profile during sodium profiling hemodialysis on the maintenance of the quality of dialysis and sodium and fluid balances. *J. Am. Soc. Nephrol.* 2005;16:237-246.

[4] Peixoto AJ, Gowda N, Parikh CR, et al. Long-term stability of serum sodium in hemodialysis patients. *Blood Purif.* 2010;29:264-267.

[5] Van der Sande FM, et al. Effect of dialysis solution calcium concentration on intradialytic blood pressure course in cardiac-compromised patients. *Am. J. Kidney Dis.* 1998; 32: 125.

[6] Lynch KE, Feldman HI, Berlin JA, et al. Effects of L-carnitine on dialysis-related hypotension and muscle cramps: a meta-analysis. *Am. J. Kidney Dis.* 2008; 52: 962-971.

[7] Hung CY, Chen YL, Chen CS, et al. Association of leptin with hemodialysis-related muscle cramps: a cross-sectional study. *Blood Purif.* 2009;27:159-164.

[8] Sherman RA, et al. Acute therapy of hemodialysis-related muscle cramps. *Am. J. Kidney Dis.* 1982;2:287–288.

[9] Kaji DM, Ackad A, Nottage WG, Stein RM. Prevention of muscle cramps in hemodialysis patients by quinine sulphate. *Lancet* 1976; ii: 66–67.

[10] Guay DR. Are there alternatives to the use of quinine to treat nocturnal leg cramps? *Consult. Pharm.* 2008;23:141-156.

[11] Ahsan M, et al. Prevention of hemodialysis-related muscle cramps by intradialytic use of sequential compression devices: a report of four cases. *Hemodial. Int.* 2004;8:283–286.

[12] Sadowski RH, Allred EN, Jabs K. Sodium modeling ameliorates intradialytic and interdialytic symptoms in young hemodialysis patients. *J. Am. Soc. Nephrol.* 1993;4:1192-1198.

[13] Arieff AI, Massry SG, Barrientos A, et al. Brain water and electrolyte metabolism in uremia: effects of slow and rapid hemodialysis. *Kidney Int.* 1973;4:177-187.

[14] Patel N, Dalal P, Panesar M. Dialysis disequilibrium syndrome: a narrative review. *Semin. Dial.* 2008;21:493-498.

[15] Ball AM, et al. Bradykinin (BK) metabolism in hemodialysis (HD): comparison of angiotensin converting enzyme inhibitors (ACEi) and angiotensin II receptor blockers (ARB). ASN Annual Meeting—San Diego. *J. Am. Soc. Nephrol.* 2003;14:712A.

[16] Hakim RM, Breillatt J, Lazarus JM, et al. Complement activation and hypersensitivity reactions to dialysis membranes. *N. Engl. J. Med.* 1984;311:878-882.

[17] Parnes EL, Shapiro WB. Anaphylactoid reactions in hemodialysis patients treated with the AN69 dialyzer. *Kidney Int.* 1991;40:1148-1152.

[18] Santoro A, Mancini E, London G, et al. Patients with complex arrhythmias during and after haemodialysis suffer from different regimens of potassium removal. *Nephrol Dial Transplant.* 2008;23:1415-1421.

[19] Bailey RA, Kaplan AA. Intradialytic cardiac arrhythmias: I. *Semin. Dial.* 1994;7:57-58.

[20] Kant KS. Intradialytic cardiac arrhythmias: II. *Semin Dial.* 1994;7: 58-60.

[21] Karnik JA, Young BS, Lew NL, et al. Cardiac arrest and sudden death in dialysis units. *Kidney Int.* 2001;60:350-357.

[22] Chazan J. Sudden deaths in patients with chronic renal failure on hemodialysis. *Dial Transplant.* 1987;16:447-448.

[23] Bleyer AJ, Russell GB, Satko SG. Sudden and cardiac death rates in hemodialysis patients. *Kidney Int.* 1999;55:1553-1559.

[24] Selby NM, McIntyre CW. The acute cardiac effects of dialysis. *Semin. Dial.* 2007;20:220-228.

[25] Gunal AL, et al. Gabapentin therapy for pruritus in hemodialysis patients:randomized placebo-controlled, double-blind trial. *Nephrol Dial Transplant* 2004;19:3137-3139.

[26] Wikstrom B, et al. Kappa-opioid system in uremic pruritus: multicenter,randomized, double-blind, placebo-controlled clinical studies. *J. Am. Soc. Nephrol.*, 2005;16:3742-3747.

[27] Cruz DN, Mahnensmith RL, Brickel HM, et al. Midodrine and cool dialysate are effective therapies for symptomatic intradialytic hypotension. *Am. J. Kidney Dis.* 1999;33:920-926.

[28] Tomson CRV. Advising dialysis patients to restrict fluid intake without restricting sodium intake is not based on evidence and is a waste of time. *Nephrol Dial Transplant* 2001;16:1538–1542.

[29] Santos SFF, et al. The consequences of an individualized dialysate Na+ prescription on hemodialysis (HD) parameters. A short-term study. ASN Annual Meeting—San Diego. *J. Am. Soc. Nephrol.* 2003;14:55A.

[30] Sherman RA, et al. Effect of variations in dialysis solution temperature on blood pressure during hemodialysis. *Am. J. Kidney Dis.* 1984;4: 66–68.

[31] Sherman RA, et al. Postprandial blood pressure changes during hemodialysis. *Am. J. Kidney Dis.* 1988;12:37–39.

[32] Strong J, et al. Effects of calorie and fluid intake on adverse events during hemodialysis. *J. Ren. Nutr.* 2001;11(2):97–100.

[33] Barakat MM, et al. Hemodynamic effects of intradialytic food ingestion and the effects of caffeine. *J. Am. Soc. Nephrol.* 1993;3:1813–1818.

[34] Santoro A, et al. Blood volume controlled hemodialysis in hypotension-prone patients: a randomized, multicenter controlled trial. *Kidney Int.* 2002;62:1034–1045.

[35] Jacob AD, Elkins N, Reiss OK, Chan L, Shapiro JI. Effects of acetate on energy metabolism and function in the isolated perfused rat heart. *Kidney Int.* 1997;52:755–760. doi: 10.1038/ki.1997.392.

[36] Canzanello VJ, Burkart JM: Hemodialysis-associated muscle cramps. *Semin. Dial.* 5:299–304, 1992.

[37] Chou CT, Wasserstein A, Schumacher HR, Fernandez P: Musculoskeletal manifestations in hemodialysis patients. *J. Rheumatol.* 12:1149–1153, 1985.
[38] Hurot JM, Cucherat M, Haugh M, Fouque D. Effect of L-carnitine supplementation in maintenance hemodialysis patients: a systematic review. *J. Am. Soc. Nephrol.* 2002;13:708–714.
[39] Ebo DG, Bosmans JL, Couttenye MM, Stevens WJ. Haemodialysis-associated anaphylactic and anaphylactoid reactions. *Allergy.* 2006;61:211–20.
[40] Schoenfeld PY. The technology of dialyzer reuse. *Semin Nephrol.* 1997 Jul;17(4):321-30.
[41] Coppo R, Amore A, Cirina P, et al. Bradykinin and nitric oxide generation by dialysis membranes can be blunted by alkaline rinsing solutions. *Kidney Int.* 2000;58:881-888.
[42] Blossom DB, Kallen AJ, Patel PR, et al. Outbreak of adverse reactions associated with contaminated heparin. *N. Engl. J. Med.* 2008;359: 2674-2684.
[43] Hakim RM, Breillatt J, Lazarus JM, et al. Complement activation and hypersensitivity reactions to dialysis membranes. *N. Engl. J. Med.* 1984;311:878-882.
[44] Jaber BL, Pereira BJG. Dialysis reactions. *Semin Dial.* 1997;10:158-165.
[45] Dialysate for Hemodialysis. Arlington: American National Standards, *Association for the Advancement of Medical Instrumentation*; 2009:1-66.
[46] Mermel LA, Allon M, Bouza E, et al. Clinical practice guidelines for the diagnosis and management of intravascular catheter-related infection: 2009 Update by the Infectious Diseases Society of America. *Clin. Infect. Dis.* 2009;49:1-45.
[47] Allon M. Treatment guidelines for dialysis catheter-related bacteremia: An update. *Am. J. Kidney Dis.* 2009;54:13-17.
[48] Sherman, Daugirdas, and Ing, 2007; Sherman, Daugirdas, and Ing, 2007.
[49] SM., S. (2011). Restless legs syndrome in patients on hemodialysis. *Saudi J. Kidney Dis. Transpl.*, 368-372.
[50] Takaki J, N. T. (2003). Clinical and psychological aspects of restless legs syndrome in uremic patients on hemodialysis. *Am. J. Kidney Dis.,* 833-839.
[51] JD, B., DM, B., A, M., 3rd, P. T., and JP., K. (1985). Uremic pruritus: skin divalent ion content and response to ultraviolet phototherapy. *American Journal of Kidney Diseases*, 5, 237-41.
[52] AI, G., G, O., TK, Y., SY, G., E, K., and H., C. (2004). Gabapentin therapy for pruritus in haemodialysis patients: a randomized, placebo-controlled, double-blind trial. *Nephrology Dialysis Transplantation*, 3137-9.
[53] Manuel MA, S. W. (1972). Air embolism during haemodialysis. *Lancet.* 538.
[54] Fan, P. Y. (1994, July). Acute vascular access: new advances. *Adv. Ren. Replace Ther.*
[55] Kwon TH, K. Y. (1997). Ultrasound-guided cannulation of the femoral vein for acute haemodialysis access. *Nephrol Dial Transplant.*, 1009-12.
[56] Wilkieson TJ, I. A. (2011). Low-intensity adjusted-dose warfarin for the prevention of hemodialysis catheter failure: a randomized, controlled trial. Clin. *J. Am. Soc. Nephrol.*, 1018-24.
[57] Macrae JM, L. G. (2005). Short and long alteplase dwells in dysfunctional hemodialysis catheters. *Hemodial Int.*, 189-95.
[58] Hemmelgarn BR, M. L.-D., and Group., P. o.-P. (2011). Prevention of dialysis catheter malfunction with recombinant tissue plasminogen activator. *N. Engl. J. Med.*, 303-312.

[59] Donati G, C. L. (2011). Thrombosis of Tunneled-Cuffed Hemodialysis Catheters: Treatment With High-Dose Urokinase Lock Therapy. *Artif. Organs.,* 1525-1594.

[60] Schwab SJ, Q. L. (1988). Hemodialysis-associated subclavian vein stenosis. *Kidney Int.* 1988, 1156-1159.

In: Hemodialysis: Indications, Procedures and Complications ISBN: 978-1-62081-301-0
Editors: Y F. Cabral and M. Costa De Santos

Chapter VI

Antiplatelet Medication and the Risk of Bleeding in Hemodialysis Patients

Shoichiro Daimon
Daimon Clinic for Internal Medicine, Nephrology and Dialysis, Ishikawa, Japan

Abstract

In hemodialysis patients, antiplatelet medications are used in various situations which include prevention of ischemic and thrombotic complications. The recent rapid increase in the number of hemodialysis patients due to diabetes mellitus and advanced age of patients has resulted in an increased demand for percutaneous intervention or coronary artery bypass grafting requiring long-term adjunctive antiplatelet or anticoagulant medications. Patients with chronic kidney disease, particularly hemodialysis patients, are at high risk of bleeding, and long-term antiplatelet therapy in hemodialysis patients may result in harmful bleeding. Despite this situation, the influence of antiplatelet therapy on bleeding in hemodialysis patients has not been sufficiently studied. We investigated bleeding events that required the cessation of the use of heparin for hemodialysis in all the hemodialysis patients treated in our clinic. During the treatment in our clinic, 21 of 52 patients with antiplatelet therapy experienced a bleeding event (gastrointestinal bleeding 16, brain stem hemorrhage 2, others 3), while 7 of 59 patients without antiplatelet therapy had a bleeding event (gastrointestinal bleeding 7) ($p<0.001$). It's worth noting that, the diabetic patients with antiplatelet therapy had the highest incidence of bleeding events. Among the patients with antiplatelet therapy, no correlations were found between bleeding events and the duration of antiplatelet therapy and the number of agents.

Our results showed that antiplatelet therapy can induce bleeding events more frequently in hemodialysis patients, especially in diabetic patients, than in non-hemodialysis patients, and antiplatelet therapy should be given only under prudent consideration of the associated risks and benefits.

Introduction

Antiplatelet medications are an important adjunctive treatment for preventing ischemic complications after percutaneous intervention (PCI) or coronary artery bypass grafting (CABG), and for preventing thrombosis in arteriosclerosis obliterans (ASO) and cerebral infarction. Although antiplatelet therapy has an associated risk of bleeding [1], the demand for treatment of cardiovascular events with these agents has been increasing because of the increase in the number of older patients and those with diabetes mellitus (DM). In general, as a treatment of cardiovascular disease, the benefits of their use outweigh the risk of bleeding [2] and the use of antiplatelet agents in this context is now well established [3-5].

Despite the fact that hemodialysis patients have been recognized to be at a high risk of bleeding [6-9], the use of antiplatelet agents in hemodialysis patients is also routine to prevent ischemic events after PCI. In hemodialysis patients, antiplatelet agents are also prescribed to prevent arteriovenous graft (AVG) thrombosis.

Since the influence of antiplatelet agents on bleeding in hemodialysis patients has not been sufficiently investigated, the use of antiplatelet agent in hemodialysis patients must be decided in individual cases based on a careful evaluation of the balance between risks and benefits in each situation.

We will discuss the influence of antiplatelet agents on non-hemodialysis and hemodialysis patients and also discuss the strategy for reducing or avoiding bleeding events observed in hemodialysis patients with antiplatelet treatment.

Antiplatelet Medications and Bleeding in Non-Hemodialysis Patients

As a defense of vascular injury, platelets adhere and aggregate at the site of injury, which makes a possible situation of arterial thrombosis after atherosclerotic plaque rupture resulting in myocardial infarction, thrombosis of ASO and cerebral infarction. Although antiplatelet therapy plays a pivotal role in preventing thrombosis, the disadvantage of this therapy is an increased risk of bleeding.

Aspirin inhibits platelet activation permanently by blocking an arachidoic cascade within the cell [10]. It is reported that for patients taking aspirin for a minimum of one year, gastrointestinal hemorrhage occurred in 2.47%, compared with 1.42% taking placebo, and that there was no correlation between aspirin dose and the incidence of gastrointestinal hemorrhage [1]. Despite this low rate of bleeding, given that more than one-third of the U.S. adults are estimated to take aspirin daily for cardiovascular disease [11], it is obvious that the substantial number of people are at risk of bleeding.

The thienopyridines (ticlopidine, clopidogrel and prasugrel) inhibit platelet activation by blocking the ADP receptor on platelets. While for patients who require PCI or CABG, the dual therapy such as aspirin and clopidogrel or the triple therapy with warfarin is recommended, in patients who require long-term prevention of thrombosis by dual or triple therapy, the risk of bleeding is much higher [12]. Compared with ticlopidine, the 1st generation thienopyridine, clopidogrel, the 2nd generation thienopyridine has a better safety profile with a lower hematologic and liver side effects. Despite the important clinical benefits, clopidogrel at approved doses has a delayed antiplatelet effect, requiring a substantial period of pretreatment for achieving the desired clinical effect. In addition, clopidogrel has a substantial inter-individual variation in its antiplatelet effect ; it is estimated that up to one third of patients have poor antiplatelet responses or resistance to clopidogrel [13-15].

Prasugrel, a novel thienopyridine, has a potent inhibitor of platelets without any low responders [16]. Although prasugrel is reported to have increased inhibition of platelets and lower risk of myocardial infarction and stent thrombosis when started at the time of PCI in patients with acute coronary syndromes, prasugrel has a higher risk of major bleeding [17].

Unlike aspirin or thienopyridines, which inactivate platelets permanently, ticagretor is a reversible and direct-acting $P2Y_{12}$ receptor antagonist, which has a greater and more constant platelet inhibition with more rapid onset and offset of action [18]. Compared with clopidogrel with aspirin, ticagretor with aspirin resulted in fewer cardiovascular death, myocardial infarction, or stroke with no different rates of PLATO-defined total major bleeding; clopidogrel with aspirin 11.6% vs ticagretor with aspirin 11.5% for 6-12 months [19].

Antiplatelet Medications and Bleeding in Hemodialysis Patients

Hemodialysis patients are at high risk of bleeding, and bleeding events, especially gastrointestinal bleeding events, are major concern under the use of antiplatelet agents. However, the effect of antiplatelet agents in hemodialysis patients has not been reported so far [20].

Clopidogrel is converted to its active form by cytochrome P450 enzymes [21] and renal impairment is not a factor of its clearance, but renal impairment can reduce the activity of these enzymes. On the other hand, ticagretor is an active, reversibly binding $P2Y_{12}$ inhibitor and renal function does not affect antiplatelet effect of ticagretor [22]. James and colleagues [23] demonstrated in the Platelet Inhibition and Patient Outcomes (PLATO) trial that ticagretor, compared with clopidogrel, significantly reduced ischemic end point and mortality in acute coronary syndrome without a significant increase in major bleeding. In their report, there was an incremental bleeding risk over the different stages of renal function. But this trial did not include patients with end-stage renal failure requiring dialysis.

Keeping with the above-mentioned problem in mind, we investigated the occurrences of bleeding events in hemodialysis patients, which required the cessation of the use of heparin in our clinic. We were also concerned with the influence of antiplatelet therapy on bleeding events [24].

Patients

All 111 patients receiving hemodialysis therapy in our clinic were investigated retrospectively. Table 1 shows the characteristics of these patients. Their mean age was 66.7 ± 11.3 years, and antiplatelet medications were used in 52 of them (female/male=15/37; age, 70.4 ± 11.3 years; number of days of hemodialysis treatment 2183 ± 2682 (31-12654) days; days of hemodialysis treatment in our clinic 1073±696 (31-2144) days; DM/non-

DM=29/23). In 59 patients antiplatelet agents were not used during treatment in our clinic (female/male, 17/42; age, 66.7 ± 14.0 years; number of days of hemodialysis treatment, 1880 ± 2110 (26-9355) days; number of days of hemodialysis treatment in our clinic, 917 ± 605 (26-2102) days; DM/non-DM, 21/28).

Except for one patient who had undergone CABG, antiplatelet therapy was administered to all patients who had undergone PCI, such as plain old balloon angioplasty (POVA; N=9), stenting (N=15)), and CABG (N=4). Vascular access interventional therapy (VAIVT) was done in 27 patients, and 14 of these 27 patients received antiplatelet therapy. Nine of 14 patients with no history of PCI were given antiplatelet medication exclusively to prevent AVG or fistula thrombosis after VAIVT, but in 5 of 14 patients the agents were instead given to prevent ischemic complications after PCI or CABG, or to prevent thrombosis of ASO and cerebral infarction.

Table 1. Patient characteristics. DM: diabetes mellitus, POBA: plan old balloon angioplasty, CABG: conorary artery bypass surgery, VAIVT: vascular access interventional therapy

	antiplatelet Yes (n=52)	antiplatelet No (n=59)	p
Age (years)	70.4±11.3	66.7±14.0	n.p.
Male	37	42	n.p.
DM	29	21	<0.05
Days of dialysis	2183(31-12654)	1880(26-9355)	n.p.
Days of dialysis in our clinic	1073(31-2144)	917(26-2102)	n.p.
POBA	9	0	<0.001
stent	15	0	0.00001
CABG	4	1	n.p.
VAIVT	14	13	n.p.
platelets (x10^4/mm^3)	18.2±5.8	17.2±5.5	n.p.
Hb (g/dL)	9.98±0.98	10.10±1.15	n.p.
Serum albumin (g/dL)	3.66±0.43	3.72±0.40	n.p.

Between patients who were or were not on antiplatelet medication, there were no statistical differences in age, days of dialysis, platelet counts, hemoglobin, or serum albumin. The proportion of diabetic patients was larger in the patients on the medication, reflecting the fact that diabetic patients are more prone to having cardiovascular disease. The number of patients and dose of antiplatelet agents are shown in Table. 2. Aspirin was the most common antiplatelet agent used. For patients with PCI, aspirin with clopidogrel or ticlopidine was used as a rule. In 3 of 4 CABG patients, warfarin was in conjunction with antiplatelet agents. A total of 3000 - 4000 units of conventional heparin is used in each session of hemodialysis.

Methods

During the hemodialysis treatment in our clinic, bleeding events that required the cessation of heparin for hemodialysis were investigated. The incidence of bleeding events in patients who were or were not have DM was compared, and the influence of the number of antiplatelets or there duration of administration on bleeding events was also investigated.

Statistics

Data were expressed as the mean ± SD. Paired t-tests and chi square test were used to compare the data. Statistical significance is defined as $P < 0.05$.

Table 2. daily dose and number of patients antiplatelet and anticoagulant medications were prescribed

	1 mg	2 mg	3 mg	25 mg	50 mg	75 mg	100 mg	150 mg	200 mg	Total
Aspirin							34		7	41
Ticlopidine							4		5	9
Clopidogrel				2	10	8				20
Cilostazol					1		2		2	5
Sarpogrelate Hydrochloride									2	2
warfarin	1	2	1							4

Results

As shown in Table 3, bleeding events were seen in 21 of 52 patients on antiplatelet therapy (40.4%), and in 7 of 59 patients not taking them (11.9%) (p<0.001). The seven bleeding events in the patients not taking them were all gastrointestinal hemorrhages (gastric cancer, *N*=2; colon cancer, *N*=1; gastric ulcer, *N*=1; acute gastric mucosal lesion, *N*=1; hemorrhagic gastritis, *N*=1; and colon polyp, *N*=1). In contrast, 16 of the 21 bleeding events in patients on antiplatelet therapy were gastrointestinal hemorrhages (gastric mucosal bleeding, *N*=4; colon polyp, *N*=3; gastric polyp, *N*=1; gastric-duodenal ulcer, *N*=1; gastric cancer, *N*=1; colon diverticula, *N*=1; ischemic colitis, *N*=1; internal hemorrhoid, *N*=1; and gastrointestinal hemorrhage of unknown origin, *N*=3) and hemoglobin dropped 0.6 g/dL to 3.4 g/dL, while 2 of 5 non-gastrointestinal hemorrhages were brain stem hemorrhages. One of these patients had been treated with warfarin and aspirin, and the other only with 100mg of aspirin under desirable blood pressure control. This patient died after 32 days after the initiation of hemodialysis. A total of 15 of 16 gastrointestinal hemorrhagic events in patients on antiplatelet therapy occurred under the use of proton pump inhibitors.

The correlation between the duration of antiplatelet use and the occurrence of bleeding events was shown in (Figure.1) No correlation was seen, with some patients receiving the medication for more than 1000 days without bleeding events, and others experiencing bleeding events within a short period of administration. Because of the small number of patients, the correlation between the dose of antiplatelet agent and bleeding events was not investigated. Regarding the patients treated with aspirin, which was used most frequently, 7 of 17 patients (41.2%) prescribed aspirin alone had bleeding events, while 10 of 24 patients (41.7%) for whom aspirin was prescribed in combination with other antiplatelet agent experienced bleeding events, suggesting that the bleeding was not dependent on the antiplatelet dosage.

Table 3. Site of bleeding events, according to antiplatelet medication

Event	Antiplatelet Yes (N=52)	Antiplatelet No (N=59)	p
Gastrointestinal bleeding	16	7	<0.05
Brain stem hemorrhage	2	0	
Retinal hemorrhage	1	0	
Vitreal hemorrhage	1	0	
AV fistula bleeding	1	0	
Total	21	7	<0.001

Table 4. Bleeding events according to antiplatelet therapy and diabetes mellitus

	Antiplatelet Yes, DM (n=29)	Antiplatelet Yes, Non-DM (n=23)	Antiplatelet No, DM (n=21)	Antiplatelet No, Non-DM (n=38)
Age (years)	68.1±11.1	73.4±11.1	66.9±10.5	66.6±15.8
Female	6	9	3	14
Days of dialysis	1475±1629	3075±3537	1110±745	2278±2552
Days of dialysis in our clinic	1068±699	1080±709	882±509	955±674
platelets ($x10^4/mm^3$)	17.5±5.5	19.1±6.1	17.0±5.8	17.5±5.4
Hb (g/dL)	10.2±1.0	9.8±0.9	10.1±0.9	10.1±1.3
Serum albumin (g/dL)	3.68±0.52	3.64±0.28	3.80±0.30	3.68±0.44
Bleeding	13(44.0%)	7(30.4%)	3(14.3%)	4(10.5%)

To investigate the influence of DM, we divided the patients into four groups:

Patients with DM receiving antiplatelet medication;
Patients without DM receiving antiplatelet medication;
Patients with DM not receiving antiplatelet medication ;
Patients without DM not receiving antiplatelet medication;

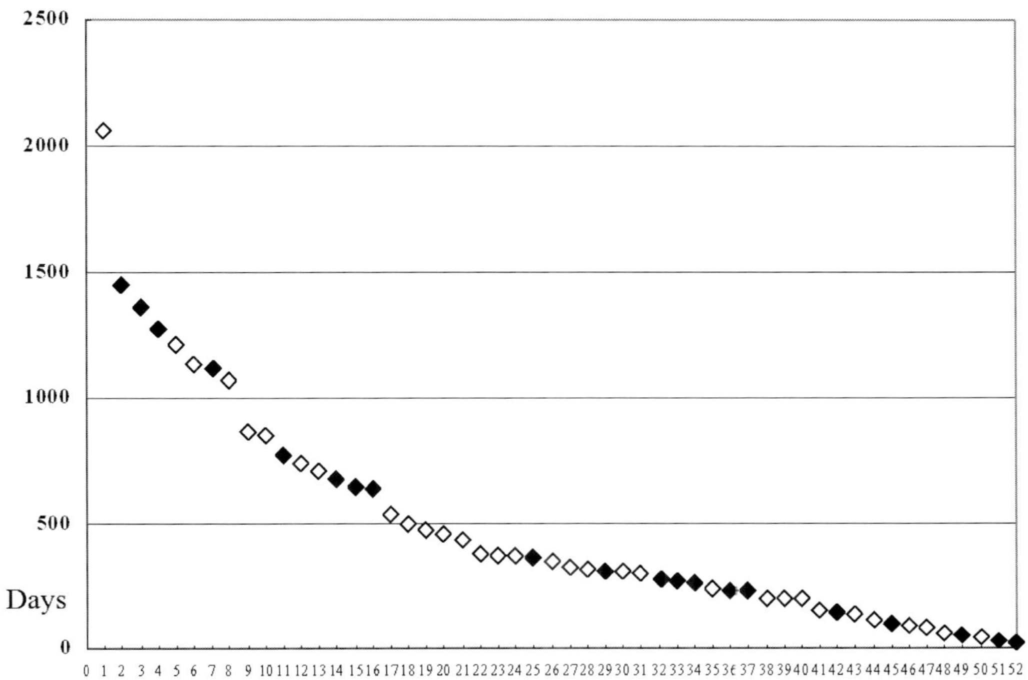

Figure 1. Days of antiplatelet medication and bleeding event : ◆Bleeding Yes (Days are from the day of start of medication to the day of Bleeding) : ◇Bleeding No.

There were no statistical differences in age, days of dialysis in our clinic, platelets counts, hemoglobin, or serum albumin levels, and bleeding events were seen in 13 of 29 (44.0%), 7 of 23 (30.4%), 3 of 21 (14.3%), and 4 of 38 (10.5%), respectively (Table 4). Statistical differences were seen between the diabetic groups with and without the antiplatelet medication (groups 1 and 3; $P<0.05$), the diabetic group on antiplatelets and the non-diabetic group without antiplatelets (groups 1 and 4; $P<0.005$), and the non-diabetic group on antiplatelets and the non-diabetic group without antiplatelets (groups 2 and 4; $P<0.05$).

Discussion

The recent rapid increase in the number of hemodialysis patients due to diabetes mellitus and advanced age of patients has resulted in an increased demand for PCI or CABG in these patients requiring long-term adjunctive antiplatelet or anticoagulant medications. Cardiovascular mortality in patients with chronic kidney disease treated by either dialysis or kidney transplantation is markedly higher than that in the general population [25], and it is reported that the prevalence of coronary artery disease at the initiation of renal replacement therapy in patients with chronic kidney disease is more than 50% notably in diabetic patients [26]. Although antiplatelet therapy in hemodialysis patients is as common as that in the general population to prevent ischemic complications after PCI or CABG, patients with end-stage renal disease are prone to develop hemostatic disorders, which might be due to platelet dysfunction, impaired platelet-vessel wall interaction, anemia, or the effect of various drugs

[6] and are regarded as being at high risk of bleeding [7-9]. The effect of antiplatelet therapy on the prevention of ischemic complications after PCI or CABG in hemodialysis patients is anticipated to be similar to that in non-hemodialysis patients, but bleeding should be kept in mind, particularly in hemodialysis patients. The risks and benefits of antiplatelet therapy in end-stage renal disease patients remaining poorly defined and the risk of a major or minor bleeding episode for hemodialysis patients was estimated to be two times and five times greater than that for non- hemodialysis patients respectively [27].

Some reports have focused on antiplatelet therapy in hemodialysis patients. Sreedhara et al reported that dipyridamole decreased the risk of thrombosis in arteriovenous graft (AVG) whereas aspirin did not [28]. But another study on the effect of clopidogrel plus aspirin on AVG thrombosis was stopped after randomization of 200 participants because of a significantly increased risk of bleeding among the participants receiving the therapy. Moreover, there was no significant benefit of active antiplatelet therapy in the prevention of thrombosis [29]. Regarding the antiplatelet therapy for hemodialysis patients with fistulas, clopidogrel was reported to reduce the frequency of early thrombosis of new arteriovenous fistulas but not to increase the proportion of patent fistulas [30]. Considering the fact that aspirin is known to increase the risk of gastrointestinal bleeding in uremic patients [31], and the indistinct anti-thrombotic effect of antiplatelet medication on AVG and fistula [28-30], the decision regarding the necessity for and the dosage of antiplatelet therapy in hemodialysis patients should be considered carefully while we weigh the balance of risks and benefits in each situation.

Our study demonstrated that antiplatelet use in hemodialysis patients resulted in an increased incidence of hemorrhage that required the cessation of heparin used for hemodialysis, most prominently in diabetic patients. We believe that this was due to vulnerability of the vessel wall in hemodialysis patients and microvascular complications associated with long-term duration of diabetes. All seven cases with bleeding in the group without antiplatelet therapy had gastrointestinal hemorrhages (gastric cancer, N=2; colon cancer, N=1; gastric ulcer, N=1; acute gastric mucosal lesion, N=1; hemorrhagic gastritis, N=1; and colon polyp, N=1), and except for the case of colon polyp, the other six cases, including the case with hemorrhagic gastritis who was a patient with liver cirrhosis, had potential causes of hemorrhage, such as cancer or an ulcer, and their bleeding events were not exclusively attributable to the uremic state. On the other hand, of the 21 cases with bleeding in the group on antiplatelet therapy, the influence of this therapy on the bleeding was considered highly marked in 15 cases (gastric mucosal bleeding, N=4; colon polyp, N=3; brain stem hemorrhage, N=2; gastric polyp, N=1; colon diverticula, N=1; retinal hemorrhage, N=1; vitreal hemorrhage, N=1; internal hemorrhoid, N=1; and ischemic colitis, N=1) because these are not common causes of bleeding in the general population and in the group without antiplatelet therapy in our study.

We could not investigate the association between the dosage of antiplatelet agent and the risk of bleeding because of the small number of patients, but of the 17 cases with receiving aspirin alone as antiplatelet therapy, seven cases (41.2%) had bleeding events, and of the 24 cases receiving aspirin as one of multiple antiplatelet agents, 10 cases (41.7%) had bleeding events, suggesting a lack of association between the dosage of antiplatelet agent and risk of bleeding. Recently, it was reported that the dose requirement of warfarin, the most commonly prescribed oral anticoagulant, should be reduced in patients with renal impairment [32]. To adjust the dosage of antiplatelet agent, there is no tool comparable to INR, which is used in patients receiving anticoagulants, and the necessity of dose adjustment of antiplatelet agents in hemodialysis patients is not yet clear. In non-hemodialysis patients, no evidence exists regarding the association between the incidence of gastrointestinal hemorrhage and the dosage of aspirin (1), and so it is not clear whether dose reduction of antiplatelet agents would be useful to reduce the incidence of bleeding in hemodialysis patients. As shown in Figure 1, some patients had bleeding events despite a short duration of antiplatelet therapy, while others had no bleeding events after prolonged use, which suggests a large patient-to-patient variability in the propensity of bleeding.

Although the benefits and outcomes of VAIVT and dialysis vascular access surgery are not clear [33], VAIVT is a familiar technique of vascular access repair in Japan, and the demand for VAIVT is increasing because of the increase in the number of hemodialysis patients with DM and/or advanced age. The effect of antiplatelet therapy after VAIVT is not clear, but considering the report that clopidogrel and aspirin did not result in a reduced frequency of AVG thrombosis and instead increased the number of bleeding events [28], antiplatelet medication after VAIVT should be avoided in general.

The increase in the number of patients with end-stage kidney disease due to the increased numbers of hemodialysis patients with DM and/or advanced age has resulted in an increased demand for PCI in hemodialysis patients. Although there is sufficient evidence to show that PCI in asymptomatic patients does not improve the survival rate in people without renal failure [34], patients of hemodialysis awaiting transplantation can benefit by screening cardiovascular angiography and PCI when significant vascular lesion exists [35]. In our clinic, if hemodialysis patients do not decline, cardiac CT or cardiovascular angiography is routine, and cardiovascular lesion is very usual. In our study, of total 111 hemodialysis patients, there were nine patients with POVA, fifteen patients with stent and four patients with CABG, but up to now only one patient died of myocardial infarction, who declined cardiovascular angiography. We believe that by applying cardio-protective strategies containing PCI or CABG, the survival rate of hemodialysis patients would improve, but as in the cases in our clinic, these strategies result in an increase in the number of hemodialysis patients with antiplatelet agents. Thus, we should keep in mind the risk of bleeding.

Although the use of drug-eluting stents has reduced the need for repeated percutaneous revascularization procedures [36, 37], early discontinuation of antiplatelet therapy after implantation of drug-eluting stents is associated with an increased incidence of thrombosis [38]. Unlike antiplatelet therapy after VAIVT, that after implantation of stents, especially drug-eluting stents, is difficult to discontinue because of the risk of cardiovascular thrombotic events. Therefore, in patients of end-stage kidney disease, especially in that with DM, cardiovascular treatments should be initiated with keeping in mind the risk of bleeding. The recent study comparing clinical outcomes following drug-eluting stents or bare-metal stents with severely reduced GFR (24% dialysis dependent) failed to demonstrate significant decrease in target-vessel revascularization and risk-adjusted rates of mortality or myocardial infarction by drug-eluting stents [39]. So, considering the high risk of bleeding, in the treatment of cardiovascular disease in hemodialysis patients, bare-metal stents, which do not necessarily require long-term antiplatelet therapy, may be more suitable than drug-eluting stents.

Long-term antiplatelet therapy in hemodialysis patients, especially in those with DM, resulted in a higher incidence of bleeding than in non-hemodialysis patients. The demand for antiplatelet therapy after PCI and CABG, or as a treatment for preventing thrombosis of ASO and cerebral infarction is increasing in hemodialysis patients. Hence, we need to devise a prudent, decision-making pathway regarding the choice of treatments and active monitoring of bleeding in those on antiplatelet therapy.

Strategies for Avoiding or Reducing Bleeding Events in Hemodialysis Patients with Antiplatelet or Anticoagulant Treatment

The possible potent strategy for avoiding or reducing gastrointestinal bleeding events in hemodialysis patients with antiplatelet agents is to use proton pump inhibitors. Proton pump inhibitors are metabolized by CYP2C19 in the liver, and clopidogrel is metabolized to its active form by several CYP isoforms, which involves CYP2C19. It is reported that proton pump inhibitors have an influence on the antiplatelet action of clopidogrel [40] and the concomitant use of clopidogrel and proton pump inhibitors was reported to be associated with an increased risk of adverse outcomes, compared with the use of clopidogrel without proton pump inhibitors [41]. Others report in clinical settings among patients receiving aspirin and clopidogrel, compared with placebo, the use of proton pump inhibitors reduce the rate of upper gastrointestinal bleeding without increasing a cardiovascular event [42]. Although the clinical influence of proton pump inhibitors on clopidogrel has been highly controversial, our study of hemodialysis patients with antiplatelet agents showed that 15 of 16 gastrointestinal hemorrhagic events in patients on antiplatelet therapy occurred under the use of proton pump inhibitors [24]. This fact suggests that the effect of proton pump inhibitors for the prevention of gastrointestinal bleeding is not so promising. Compared with aspirin, thienopyridines (ticlopidine and clopidogrel) are reported to have less gastrointestinal hemorrhage [43, 44], so if a single antiplatelet therapy is possible, thienopyridine rather than aspirin may be a better choice.

On the other hand, in regard of intracranial and extracranial hemorrhage, aspirin and thienopiyridines are reported to have comparable risks [43], and the risk of hemorrhagic stroke, which is small in healthy individuals, is surprisingly high in hemodialysis patients and is associated with high mortality [45]. In our present study, two of 52 patients with antiplatelet therapy died of brain stem hemorrhages, which were not seen in patients without antiplatelet therapy, suggesting an association between antiplatelet therapy and hemorrhagic stroke in hemodialysis patients.

Cilostazol is a unique antiplatelet agent. Unlike other antiplatelet agents, cilostazol not only inhibits platelet function but also improves vascular endothelial cell function and may reduce the risk of stroke without increasing the risk of bleeding complications [46]. Cilostazol is reported to be superior to aspirin for prevention of stroke and was associated with fewer hemorrhagic events [47], and was as effective as ticlopidine [48, 49] or clopidogrel [50] in preventing stent thrombosis after coronary stent placement with a comparable rate of side effects which include bleeding. Another potential benefit of the use of cilostazol is the short recovery time (12-16 hours) of platelet function [51]. Although the advantages and disadvantages of cilostazol over the other antiplatelet agents in hemodialysis patients are not known, cilostazol alone or with other antiplatelet agents may be one option as a long-term adjunctive therapy for the prevention of thrombosis with fewer bleeding events.

In addition, we should notice that, not only antiplatelet agents, but anticoagulant agents may also be the cause of bleeding in hemodialysis patients. It is reported recently that in older hemodialysis patients with atrial fibrillation, compared with non-users, warfarin users had twice the risk of hemorrhagic stroke with the comparable risks of ischemic stroke, gastrointestinal hemorrhage, and mortality [52]. Like proton pump inhibitors, warfarin is primarily metabolized by the hepatic CYP450 system. In end-stage renal disease, hepatic CYP450 metabolism is downregulated [53], and renal impairment can affect the pharmacokinetics of drugs that are predominantly eliminated by nonrenal processes [54]. Dose requirement of warfarin is reported to be reduced in patients with renal impairment [32], which we should keep in mind whenever we use warfarin in hemodialysis patients.

Conclusion

To summarize, although further study is needed to confirm the relationship between antiplatelet therapy and bleeding events in hemodialysis patients, our study demonstrated that the risk bleeding due to antiplatelet therapy in hemodialysis patients is high compared with non-hemodialysis patients, especially in diabetic patients. Although we have several options of antiplatelet agents available, currently reliable information about benefits and risks of each antiplatelet agent in hemodialysis patients is scarce. In order to respond the increasing demand for antiplatelet therapy after PCI and CABG, or as a treatment for preventing thrombosis of ASO and cerebral infarction in hemodialysis patients, the decision about whether and how to use antiplatelet agents in hemodialysis patients should be made cautiously depending on individual cases based on a careful evaluation of the balance of risks and benefits.

References

[1] Derry S and Loke YK. Risk of gastrointestinal haemorrhage with long term-use of aspirin: meta analysis. *BMJ* 2000; 321: 1183-1187.

[2] Steinhubl SR, Bhatt DL, Brennan BM, et al. Aspirin to prevent cardiovascular disease: the association of aspirin dose and clopidogrel with thrombosis and bleeding. *Ann Intern Med* 2009; 150: 379-386.

[3] Leon MB, Baim DS, Popma JJ, et al. A clinical trial comparing three antithrombotic-drug regimens after coronary-artery stenting. N Engl J *Med* 1998; 339: 1665-1671.

[4] Mehta SR, Yusuf S, Peters RJG, et al. Effects of pretreatment with clopidogrel and aspirin followed by long-term therapy in patients undergoing percutaneous coronary intervention: the PCI-CURE study. *Lancet* 2001; 358: 527-533.

[5] Bhatt DL, Fox KAA, Hacke W, et al. Clopidogrel and aspirin versus aspirin alone for the prevention of atherothrombotic events. N Engl J *Med* 2006; 354: 1706-1717.

[6] Kaw D and Malhotra D. Platelet dysfunction and end-stage renal disease. *Semin Dial* 2006; 19: 317-322.

[7] P.K.B. Jaminidar In: AR FRGD Nissenson, Editor, Gastrointestinal disease in patients with chronic renal failure. Chapter 26 in clinical dialysis vol. 3, East Norwalk, Appleton and Lange, 1995; pp. 607-617.

[8] Iseki K, Kinjo K, Kimura Y, et al. Evidence for high risk of cerebral haemorrhage in chronic dialysis patients. *Kidney Int* 1993; 44: 1086-1090.

[9] Lohr J, Schwab S. Minimizing hemorrhagic complications in dialysis patients. *J Am Soc Nephrol* 1991; 2: 961-975.

[10] Patrono C. Aspirin as an antiplatelet drug. N Engl J *Med* 1994; 330: 1287-1294.

[11] Ajani UA, Ford ES, Greenland KJ, et al. Aspirin use among U.S. adults: Behavioral risk factor surveillance system. Am J *Prev Med* 2006; 30: 74-77.

[12] Hansen M, Sørensen R, Clausen MT, et al. Risk of bleeding with single, dual, or triple therapy with warfarin, aspirin, and clopidogrel in patients with atrial fibrillation. *Arch Intern Med* 2010; 170: 1433-1441.

[13] Gurbel PA, Bliden KP, Hiatt BL, O'Connor CM. Clopidogrel for coronary stenting: Response variability, drug resistance, and the effect of pretreatment platelet reactivity. *Circulation* 2003; 107: 2908-2913.

[14] Serebruany VL, Steinhubl SR, Berger PB, et al. Variability in platelet responsiveness to clopidogrel among 544 individuals. J *Am Coll Cardiol* 2005; 45: 246-251.

[15] Wiviott SD. Clopidogrel response variability, resistance, or both? *Am J Cardiol* 2006; 98: 18N-24N.

[16] Wiviott SD, Trenk D, Frelinger AL, et al. Prasugrel compared with high loading- and maintenance-dose clopidogrel in patients with planned percutaneous coronary intervention: the Prasugrel in Comparison to Clopidogrel for Inhibition of Platelet Activation and Aggregation-Thrombolysis in Myocardial Infarction 44 trial. *Circulation* 2007; 116: 2923-2932.

[17] Wiviott SD, Braunwald E, McCabe CH, et al. Prasugrel versus clopidogrel in patients with acute coronary syndromes. N Engl J *Med* 2007; 357: 2001-2015.

[18] Gurbel PA, Bliden KP, Butler K, et al. Randomized double-blind assessment of the ONSET and OFFSET of the antiplatelet effects of ticagretor versus clopidogrel in patients with stable coronary artery disease: the ONSET/OFFSET study. *Circulation* 2009; 120: 2577-2585.

[19] Cannon CP, Harrington RA, James S, et al. Comparison of ticagretor with clopidogrel in patients with a planned invasive strategy for acute coronary syndromes (PLATO): a randomized double-blind study. *Lancet* 2010; 375: 283-292.

[20] Alexander P, David S and McCullough PA. Drug-eluting coronary stent in patients with kidney disease. Am J *Kidney Dis* 2011; 57(2): 188-189.

[21] Tang M, Mukundan M, Yang J, et al. Antiplatelet agents aspirin and clopidogrel are hydrolyzed by distinct carboxylesterases, and clopidogrel is transesterificated in the presence of ethyl alcohol. J *Pharmacol Exp Ther* 2006; 319: 1467-1476.

[22] Montalescot G and Silvain J. Ticagretor in the renal dysfunction subgroup: subjugated or substantiated? *Circulation* 2010; 122: 1049-1052.

[23] James S, Budaj A, Aylward P, et al. Ticagretor versus clopidogrel in acute coronary syndromes in relation to renal function. *Circulation* 2010; 122: 1056-1067.

[24] Daimon S and Terai H. Influence of antiplatelet medications on bleeding events in hemodialysis patients. *Ther Apher Dial*, 2011; 15(5) 454-9.

[25] Dennis VW. Coronary heart disease in patients with chronic kidney disease. J *Am Soc Nephrol* 2005; 16: S103-106.

[26] Ohtake T, Kobayashi S, Moriya H, et al. High prevalence of occult coronary artery stenosis in patients with chronic kidney disease at the initiation of renal replacement therapy: an angiographic examination. J *Am Soc Nephrol* 2005; 16: 1141-1148.

[27] Hiremath S, Holden RM, Fergusson D, et al. Antiplatelet medications in hemodialysis patients: A systemic review of bleeding rates. *Clin J Am Soc Nephrol* 2009; 4: 1347-1355.

[28] Sreedhara R, Himmelfarb J, Azarus J, Hakim R. Antiplatelet therapy in expanded polytetrafluoroethylene (ePTEE) graft thrombosis: Results of a prospective, randomized double-blind study. Kidney Int 1994; 45: 1477-1483.

[29] Kaufman JS, O'connor TZ, Zhang JH, et al. Randomized controlled trial of clopidogrel plus aspirin to prevent hemodialysis access thrombosis. J *Am Soc Nephrol* 2003; 14: 2313-2321.

[30] Dember LM, Beck GJ, Allon M, et al. for the Dialysis Access Consortium Study Group. Effect of clopidogrel on early failure of arteriovenous fistulas for hemodialysis. *JAMA* 2008; 299(18): 2164-2171.

[31] Livio M, Benigni A, Vigano G, et al. Moderate doses of aspirin and risk of bleeding in renal failure. *Lancet* 1986; 1: 414-416.

[32] Limdi NA, Limdi MA, Cavallari L, et al. Warfarin dosing in patients with impaired kidney function. Am J *Kidney Dis* 2010; 56: 823-831.

[33] Tordoir JH, Bode AS, Peppelenbosch N, et al. Surgical or endovascular repair of thrombosed dialysis vascular access: is there any evidence? J *Vasc Surg* 2009; 50: 953-956.

[34] McFalls EO, Ward HB, Moritz TE, et al. Coronary-artery revascularization before elective major vascular surgery. N Engl J *Med* 2004; 351: 2795-2804.

[35] Kumar N, Baker CSR, Chan K, et al. Cardiac survival after pre-emptive coronary angiography in transplant patients and those awaiting transplantation. Clin J *Am Soc Nephrol* 2011; 6: 1912-1919.

[36] Moses JW, Leon MB, Popma JJ, et al. Sirolimus-eluting stents versus standard stents in patients with stenosis in a native coronary artery disease. N Engl J *Med* 2003; 349: 1315-1323.

[37] Stone GW, Ellis SG, Cox DA, et al. A polymer-based, paclitaxel-eluting stent in patients with coronary artery disease. N Engl J *Med* 2004; 350: 221-231

[38] Iakovou I, Schmidt T, Bonizzoni E, et al. Incidence, predictors, and outcome of thrombosis after successful implantation of drug-eluting stents. *JAMA* 2005; 293: 2126-2130

[39] Charytan DM, Varma MR, Silbaugh TS, et al. Long-term clinical outcomes following drug-eluting or bare-metal stent placement in patients with severely reduced GFR: results of the Massachusetts Data Analysis Center (Mass-DAC) study registry. Am J *Kidney Dis* 2011; 57(2): 202-211.

[40] Gilard M, Arnaud B, Cornily JC, et al. Influence of omeprazole on the antiplatelet action of clopidogrel associated with aspirin. J *Am Coll Cardiol* 2008; 51: 256-260.

[41] Ho PM, Maddox TM, Wang L, et al. Risk of adverse outcomes associated with concomitant use of clopidogrel and proton pump inhibitors following acute coronary syndrome. *JAMA* 2009; 301(9): 937-944.

[42] Bhatt DL, Cryer BL, Contant CF, et al. Clopidogrel with or without omeprazole in coronary artery disease. N Engl J *Med* 2010; 363: 1909-1917.

[43] Hankey GJ, Sudlow CLM, and Dunbabin DW. Thienopyridines or aspirin to prevent stroke and other serious vascular events in patients at high risk of vascular disease? : a systematic review of the evidence from randomized trials. *Stroke* 2000; 31: 1779-1784.

[44] Maurice JB, Wedderburn CJ, Mason G, et al. Thienopyridine devivatives versus aspirin for preventing stroke and other serious vascular events in high vascular risk patients. *Stroke* 2010; 41: e457-e459.

[45] Power A, Chan K, Singh SK, et al. Appraising stroke risk in maintenance hemodialysis patients: a large single-center cohort study. Am J *Kidney Dis* 2011 Sep 26 (Epub ahead of print).

[46] Goto S. Cilostazol: potential mechanism of action for antithrombotic effects accompanied by a low rate of bleeding. *Atheroscler Suppl* 2005; 6(4): 3-11.

[47] Shinohara Y, Katayama Y, Uchiyama S, et al. Cilostazol for prevention of secondary stroke (CSPS 2): as aspirin-controlled, double-blind, randomized non-inferiority trial. *Lancet Neurol* 2010; 9: 959-968.

[48] Park SW, Lee CW, Kim HS, et al. Comparison of cilostazol versus ticlopidine therapy after stent implantation. Am J *Cardiol* 1999; 84: 511-514.

[49] Yoon Y, Shim WH, Lee DH, et al. Usefulness of cilostazol versus ticlopidine in coronary artery stenting. Am J *Cardiol* 1999; 84: 1375-1380.

[50] Lee SW, Park SW, Hong MK, et al. Comparison of cilostazol and clopidogrel after successful coronary stenting. Am J *Cardiol* 2005; 95: 859-862.

[51] Iwamoto T, Kin K, Miyazaki K, et al. Recovery of platelet function after withdrawal of cilostazol administered orally for a long period. *J Atheroscler Thromb* 2003; 10: 348-354.

[52] Winkelmayer WC, Liu J, Setoguchi S, et al. Effectiveness and safety of warfarion initiation in older hemodialysis patients with incident atrial fibrillation. Clin J *Am Soc Nephrol* 2011; 6: 2662-2668.

[53] Leblond F, Guevin C, Demers C, et al. Downregulation of hepatic cytochrome P450 in chronic renal failure. J *Am Soc Nephrol* 2001; 12(2): 326-332.

[54] Zhang Y, Zhang L, Abraham S, et al. Assessment of the impact of renal impairment on systemic exposure of new molecular entities: evaluation of recent new drug application. *Clin Pharmacol Ther* 2009; 85(3): 305-311.

In: Hemodialysis: Indications, Procedures and Complications ISBN: 978-1-62081-301-0
Editors: Y F. Cabral and M. Costa De Santos

Chapter VII

Vascular Calcifications in End Stage Renal Disease

Lucia Di Micco, Francesco Mirenghi, Maria Luisa Sirico, Serena Torraca and Biagio Di Iorio
UOC of Nephrology, "Agostino Landolfi" Hospital, ASL Avellino, Solofra, Italy

Abstract

Vascular calcifications (VCs) are more frequent and severe in patients with CKD on dialysis than in subjects from the general population. Both high phosphorus and positive calcium balance from calcium-containing phosphate binders are considered as strong responsible factors of vascular calcification process and adverse events. Therefore, guidelines recommend limiting the use of calcium containing phosphate binders in presence of known vascular and or valvular calcifications in CKD patients not yet on dialysis. We describe our experience on vascular calcification in dialysis patients. These results indicated that CAC could represent a step in the continuum of events responsible for the CV mortality in CKD-5.

Keywords: Vascular calcification, hemodialysis, ESRD

Introduction

Over the past 10 years a great amount of literature has been produced to study the relationship between serum levels of bone minerals, vitamin D, intact parathyroid hormone (iPTH), the cardiovascular (CV) system, and mortality. These associations were first studied in patients on dialysis [1-3], and then they were confirmed in chronic kidney disease (CKD) patients not requiring dialysis [4], and in people with normal renal function [5-8]. Nonetheless, despite a huge quantity of data on the existing association between serum phosphorus levels and all-cause mortality in dialysis patients [2,3], only few studies evaluated the adverse effects of hyperphosphatemia on renal function and prognosis in CKD subjects [9-14].In the general population, vascular calcifications are a consequence of the atherosclerotic disease and of the natural history of atherosclerotic plaques. Vascular calcifications (VCs) and particularly coronary artery calcifications (CAC) are more frequent and severe in patients with CKD on dialysis than in subjects from the general population [15-19]. In addition, VCs are strongly associated with CV events such as myocardial infarction, symptomatic angina pectoris, and stroke [16,17,19-21].CAC have been found nearly in a half of patients with early stages of CKD [22-24]; in presence of diabetes, the number of patients with VC was even higher [24-26].VCs in CKD patients are different from those of non-uremic subjects, in which they are located in the endothelium. On the other side, VCs of uremic patients are located in the media layer of arterial wall of vessels of any size, including arterioles, determining arterial stiffness and deteriorating the elastic properties of vessels. As the atherosclerotic process leading to VCs is a continuum from early stages of CKD to dialysis, it is likely that VCs in CKD patients not yet on dialysis have similar location (both in intimal and media layer of arterial wall), and cause similar hemodynamic changes to those observed in patients on dialysis [16,17,21].Although the clinical importance of VCs and particularly of CAC has been recognized for long time, there are no studies evaluating whether intervention that potentially may dampen VCs improves outcomes in CKD patients not requiring dialysis. In fact, few studies have been performed in this population and only aimed to evaluate the effects of either statins or different phosphate binders on progression of CAC; a slower progression of CAC was observed in patients treated with statins compared to controls [27,28] and in patients treated with sevelamer compared to those treated with calcium carbonate [29]. Both high phosphorus and positive calcium balance from calcium-containing phosphate binders are considered as strong responsible factors of vascular calcification process and adverse events. Therefore, guidelines recommend limiting the use of calcium containing phosphate binders in presence of known vascular and or valvular calcifications in CKD patients not yet on dialysis [30,31].

Our Experience in Dialysis Patients

In a previous paper we reported an independent association between CAC and electrocardiogram (ECG) abnormalities (i.e. QT dispersion (QTd), suggesting that VC may affect cardiac repolarization and may predispose to cardiac arrhythmia [32]. To evaluate prospectively the association between VCs and outcomes we performed the Independent study [33], a randomized controlled trial designed to investigate the impact of two different phosphate binder regimes (sevelamer HCl vs. calcium or aluminium salts) on mortality in hemodialysis patients, we analysed the hypothesis that CAC progression was linked to an increase in arterial stiffness and cardiac repolarization abnormalities. Inclusion criteria were a history of CKD requiring dialysis for <120 days. Exclusion criteria included age >75 years, concomitant acute illness or history of cardiac arrhythmia, history of coronary artery bypass, liver dysfunction and hypothyroidism and use of drugs that prolong the QT interval. CAC score (CACS), PWV and QTd were evaluated at study entry and after 12 months. CACS was assessed by a multislice light-speed (GE Medical Systems) equipment at one center (Solofra, Italy). We enrolled 466 patients. The study cohort consisted of middle-aged (65.3±16.6 years) subjects (64% men and 36% women). As expected, diabetes (23% of the entire study cohort), arterial hypertension (79.5%), and ASCVD (34%) were the most common comorbidities recorded. At dialysis entry, 70% of patients showed evidence of CAC. Specifically, 26%, 11% and 33% exhibited an Agatston CACS of 0–100, 100–400 and > 400, respectively. A true progression of CAC was detected in 61% patients. Progressors were on average older ($p<0.001$) and more likely to be diabetic ($p<0.001$). They had a greater burden of coronary artery disease and higher levels of serum C-Reactive Protein (CRP) at baseline. Instead, at study completion, progressors exhibited lower levels of serum albumin and a less favorable mineral metabolism control. A significantly greater proportion of non-progressors were treated with sevelamer HCl when compared to progressors (75 vs. 20%, $p<0.001$). During the study follow-up there was no difference in blood pressure, anemia, acidosis, diabetes lipid and mineral metabolism control between progressors and non-progressors (data not shown). After adjustment for risk factors, CAC progression was independently associated with diabetes (odds ratio (OR) diabetes vs. non-diabetes 1.17; 95% CI 1.13–1.28; $p = 0.01$), serum LDL cholesterol (OR per 10-mg/dl increase 1.07; 95% CI 1.01–1.12; $p = 0.05$), serum CRP (OR per 5-mg/dl increase 1.09; 95% CI 1.04–1.18; $p = 0.05$), use of sevelamer HCl (OR 0.66; 95% CI 0.36–0.81; $p < 0.001$). A significant change in CAC burden was associated with changes in arterial stiffness and cardiac repolarization. Although there was no difference in PWV and QTcd between groups at baseline, CAC progression was associated with a significantly greater increase in PWV and QTd at study completion. A significant increase in arterial stiffness was noted among progressors but not among non-progressors (PWV increased from 8.8±1.7 to 11.0±2.7 m/s, $p< 0.05$, and from 7.5±1.9 to 8.7±2.0 m/s, p = NS, in progressors and non-progressors, respectively). Multivariable analyses confirmed the independent associations of CAC progression with changes in PWV and QTd. Specifically, after adjustment for confounders, every 20-unit increase of CAC corresponded to a significant 23% (95% CI 1.12–1.27; $p<0.001$) and 32% (95% CI 1.09–1.37; $p<0.01$) increase in the risk of experiencing a 1-m/s increase in PWV and 1 ms in QTd, respectively. Figure 1 shows the risk of death in progressor and in non- progressor patients (log-rank test= 25.8; $p<0.0001$); when we analysed the risk of death of patients distributed for quartiles of CAC, we showed that the first quartile had a risk of 0, with a significant increase for successive quartiles (log-rank test = 57.1; $p<0.0001$) (figure 2).

Our study provided evidence of the close association of functional and morphological vascular disease markers. Patients experiencing CAC progression were at significantly greater risk of experiencing a simultaneous deterioration of markers of arterial compliance and cardiac repolarization. These results indicated that CAC could represent a step in the continuum of events responsible for the CV mortality in CKD-5 [34].

Conclusion

An excellent control of the bone metabolism with good biomechanical properties is of paramount importance in CKD patients. CKD-related bone disorder has been defined as the systemic disorder of mineral and bone metabolism characterized by one or more of the following: abnormalities of calcium, phosphorus, parathyroid hormone, or vitamin D metabolism; abnormalities in bone turnover, mineralization, volume, linear growth, or strength; and vascular or other soft tissue calcifications [35].

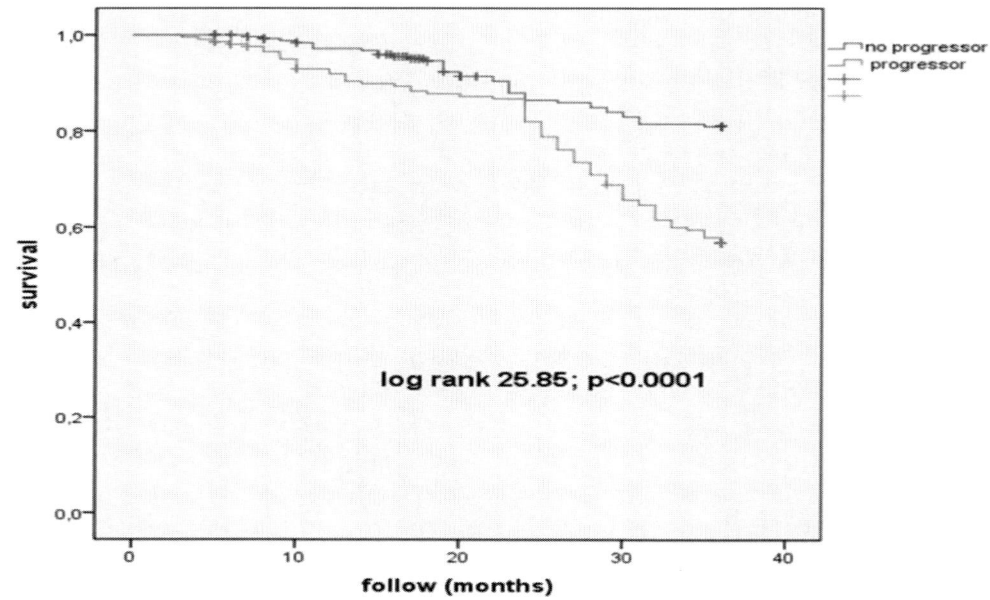

Figure 1. Survival in progressor and non-progressor patients.

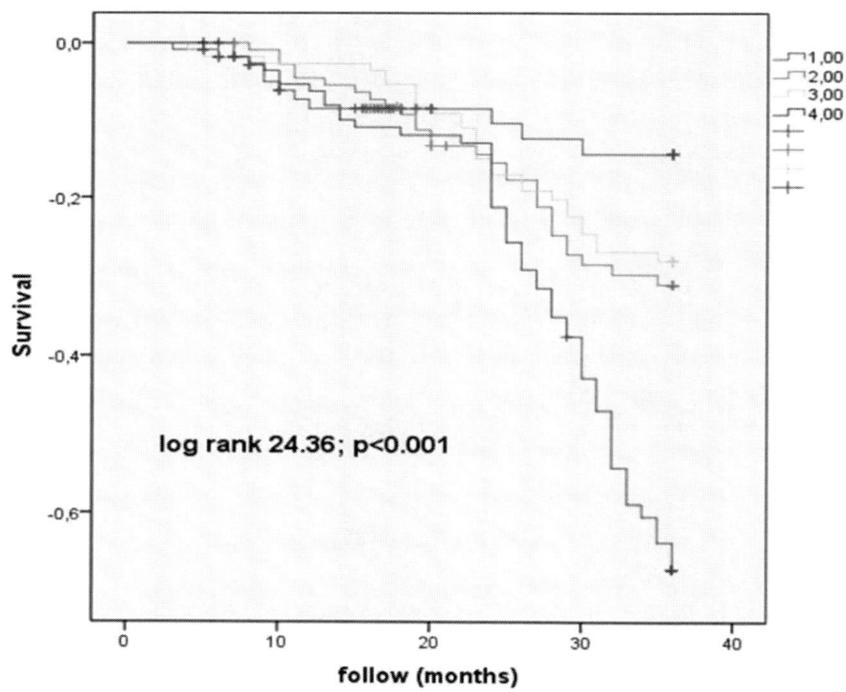

Figure 2. Survival in quartiles of vascular calcification.

Hyperphosphatemia is one of the most common metabolic complications of ESRD [1,2]. Large observational studies identified hyperphosphatemia as an independent risk factor for CV disease and mortality in dialysis, and also very small increases in serum phosphate levels within the normal range were found to be associated with a high risk of death in CKD not requiring dialysis and even in not renal disease populations. Consequently, current national practice guidelines recommend more intensive treatment of hyperphosphatemia in order to lower serum phosphate levels more than nephrologists aimed in the past. A dietary phosphorus intake restriction is recommended, but as it is difficult to obtain and maintain and it can exacerbate protein malnutrition, administration of phosphorus binders to reduce intestinal phosphorus absorption is a key point in the therapy of hyperphosphatemia [36].

The relationship between hyperphosphatemia and adverse outcomes in dialysis patients suggests that lowering serum phosphate levels may improve clinical outcomes [37]. Phosphate plays a central role in the pathophysiology of CKD-MBD and the progression of CKD and contributes to increase the CV risk of CKD patients. In fact, it has been shown that, even in early CKD stages, high levels of phosphorus promote vascular calcification, hypertension, myocardial hypertrophy and heart failure. CAC progression is a key point for mortality and morbidity in CKD and dialysis patients. Renal failure increases the extent of calcification in atherosclerotic plaques, and its effect on medial calcification is probably greater. In fact it rarely occurs in individuals without renal insufficiency under the age of 60 years [32], whereas CAC scores are almost 3 times greater in ESRD patients than in age- and sex-matched general population. In unselected autopsy cases, the prevalence of calcified coronary plaques was 52% in 27 patients with CKD compared with 37% in 30 subjects without CKD [40]. The morbidity of atherosclerosis is due to vascular occlusion, but it is unclear whether this is exacerbated by plaque calcifications. The reduction of arterial dispensability and compliance may transmit a greater pulse pressure to the distal arteries, leading to vascular insufficiency, stiffness and tissue damage through arteriolosclerosis [40]. A number of studies showed that arterial calcification and progression of calcifications correlate with cardiovascular events or mortality, and with hemodynamic parameters, such as pulse wave velocity. A study including incident hemodialysis patients found that treatment with calcium-containing phosphate binders induced a reduction of mortality associated to a reduced progression of CAC, suggesting a beneficial effect of treating vascular calcification [1-2, 41-42].

References

[1] Block GA, Hulbert-Shearon TE, Levin NW, Port FK: Association of serum phosphorus and calcium x phosphate product with mortality risk in chronic hemodialysis patients: A national study. *Am. J. Kidney Dis.*, 31: 607–617, 1998.

[2] Block GA, Klassen PS, Lazarus JM, Ofsthun N, Lowrie EG, Chertow GM: Mineral metabolism, mortality, and morbidity in maintenance hemodialysis. *J. Am. Soc. Nephrol.*, 15: 2208–2218, 2004.

[3] Kalantar-Zadeh K, Kuwae N, Regidor DL, Kovesdy CP, Kilpatrick RD, Shinaberger CS, McAllister CJ, Budoff MJ, Salusky IB, Kopple JD: Survival predictability of time-

varying indicators of bone disease in maintenance hemodialysis patients. Kidney Int 70: 771–780, 2006.

[4] Kestenbaum B, Sampson JN, Rudser KD, Patterson DJ, Seliger SL, Young B, Sherrard DJ,Andress DL: Serum phosphate levels and mortality risk among people with chronic kidney disease. *J. Am. Soc. Nephrol.*, 16: 520–528, 2005.

[5] Dhingra R, Sullivan LM, Fox CS, Wang TJ, D'Agostino RB, Sr., Gaziano JM, Vasan RS: Relations of serum phosphorus and calcium levels to the incidence of cardiovascular disease in the community. *Arch. Intern. Med.*, 167: 879–885, 2007.

[6] Onufrak SJ, Bellasi A, Cardarelli F, Vaccarino V, Muntner P, Shaw LJ, Raggi P: Investigation of gender heterogeneity in the associations of serum phosphorus with incident coronary artery disease and all-cause mortality. *Am. J. Epidemiol.*, 169: 67–77, 2009.

[7] Tonelli M, Sacks F, Pfeffer M, Gao Z, Curhan G: Relation between serum phosphate level and cardiovascular event rate in people with coronary disease. *Circulation*, 112: 2627–2633, 2005.

[8] Foley RN, Collins AJ, Herzog CA, Ishani A, Kalra PA: Serum phosphorus levels associate with coronary atherosclerosis in young adults. *J. Am. Soc. Nephrol.*, 20: 397–404, 2009.

[9] Voormolen N, Noordzij M, Grootendorst DC, Beetz I, Sijpkens YW, van Manen JG, Boeschoten EW, Huisman RM, Krediet RT, Dekker FW: High plasma phosphate as a risk factor for decline in renal function and mortality in pre-dialysis patients. *Nephrol. Dial. Transplant.*, 22: 2909–2916, 2007.

[10] Kovesdy CP, Ahmadzadeh S, Anderson JE, Kalantar-Zadeh K: Secondary hyperparathyroidism is associated with higher mortality in men with moderate to severe chronic kidney disease. *Kidney Int.*, 73: 1296–1302, 2008.

[11] Schwarz S, Trivedi BK, Kalantar-Zadeh K, Kovesdy CP: Association of disorders in mineral metabolism with progression of chronic kidney disease. *Clin. J. Am. Soc. Nephrol.*, 1: 825–831,2006.

[12] Norris KC, Greene T, Kopple J, Lea J, Lewis J, Lipkowitz M, Miller P, Richardson A, Rostand S, Wang X, Appel LJ: Baseline predictors of renal disease progression in the African American Study of Hypertension and Kidney Disease. *J. Am. Soc. Nephrol.*, 17: 2928–2936, 2006.

[13] Kovesdy CP, Anderson JE, Kalantar-Zadeh K: Outcomes associated with serum phosphorus level in males with non-dialysis dependent chronic kidney disease. *Clin. Nephrol.*, 73:268–275, 2010.

[14] Menon V, Greene T, Pereira AA, Wang X, Beck GJ, Kusek JW, Collins AJ, Levey AS, Sarnak MJ: Relationship of phosphorus and calcium-phosphorus product with mortality in CKD. *Am. J. Kidney Dis.*, 46: 455–463, 2005.

[15] Braun J, Oldendorf M, Moshage W, et al. Electron beam computed tomography in the evaluation of cardiac calcification in chronic dialysis patients. *Am. J. Kidney Dis.*, 1996; 27: 394-401.

[16] Raggi P, Boulay A, Chasan-Taber S, et al. Cardiac calcification in adult hemodialysis patients. A link between end-stage renal disease and cardiovascular disease? *JACC*, 2002; 39:695-701.

[17] Goldsmith D, Ritz E, Covic A. Vascular calcification: a stiff challenge for the nephrologists. *Kidney Int.*, 2004; 66:1315-1333.

[18] Chertow GM, Burke SK, Raggi P: Sevelamer attenuates the progression of coronary and aortic calcification in hemodialysis patients. *Kidney Int.*, 2002; 62:245-252.

[19] Coen G, Pierantozzi A, Spizzichino D, et al. Risk factors of one year increment of coronary calcifications and survival in hemodialysis patients. *BMC Nephrology*, 2010; 11:1-9.

[20] Sarnak JM. Cardiovascular complications in chronic kidney disease. *Am. J. Kidney Dis.*, 2003; 41:S11-S17.

[21] London GM. Cardiovascular calcifications in uremic patients: clinical impact on cardiovascular function. *J. Am. Soc. Nephrol.*, 2003; 14:S305-309.

[22] Russo D, Palmiero G, De Blasio AP, et al. Coronary artery calcification in patients with CRF not undergoing dialysis. *Am. J. Kidney Dis.*, 2004, 44: 1024– 1030.

[23] Russo D, Corrao S, Miranda I, et al. Progression of coronary artery calcification in predialysis patients. *Am. J. Nephrol.*, 2007; 152–158.

[24] Kramer H, Toto R, Peshock R, et al. Association between chronic kidney disease and coronary artery calcification: The Dallas Heart Study. *J. Am. Soc. Nephrol.*, 2005; 16: 507–513.

[25] Chiu YW, Adler SG, Budoff MJ, et al. Coronary artery calcification and mortality in diabetic patients with proteinuria. *Kidney Int.*, 2010; 77:1107-1114.

[26] Merjanian R, Budoff M, Adler S, et al. Coronary artery, aortic wall, and valvular calcification in non dialyzed individuals with type 2 diabetes and renal disease. *Kidney Int.*, 2003;64:263-271.

[27] Callister TQ, Raggi P, Cooil B, et al. Effect of HMG-CoA reductase inhibitors on coronary artery diseaseas assessed by electron-beam computed tomography. *N. Engl. J. Med.*, 1998;339: 1972–1978.

[28] Achenbach S, Ropers D, Pohle K, et al. Influence of lipid-lowering therapy on the progression of coronary artery calcification: A prospective evaluation. *Circulation*, 2002;106: 1077–1082.

[29] Russo D, Miranda I, Ruocco C, et al. The progression of coronary artery calcification in pre-dialysis patients on calcium carbonate or sevelamer. *Kidney Int.*, 2007; 2: 1255–1261.

[30] National Kidney Foundation. K/DOQI clinical practice guidelines for bone metabolism and disease in chronic kidney disease. *Am. J. Kidney Dis.*, 2003; 42: S1–20.

[31] KDIGO: Clinical Practice Guideline For The Diagnosis, Evaluation, Prevention, and Treatment of Chronic Kidney Disease-Mineral and Bone Disorder (CKD-MBD). *Kidney Int.*, 2009;76:S1-S130.

[32] Di Iorio BR, Bortone S, Piscopo C, Grimaldi P, Cucciniello E, D'Avanzo E, Mondillo F, Cillo N, Bellizzi V: Cardiac vascular calcification and QT interval in ESRD patients: is there a link? *Blood Purif.*, 2006; 24: 451–459.

[33] Di Iorio BR, Cucciniello E, Bellizzi V: Vascular calcification and QT interval in incident hemodialysis patients. *J. Nephrol.*, 2009; 22:694–698.

[34] Di Iorio B, Nargi O, Cucciniello V, Bellizzi V, Torraca V, Russo D, Bellasi A: Coronary artery Calcification Progression is Associated with Arterial Stiffness and Cardiac Repolarization Deterioration in Hemodialysis Patients.

[35] Confavreux CB: Bone: from a reservoir of minerals to a regulator of energy metabolism. *Kidney Int.*, 2011;79 (S121):14-19.

[36] Isakova T, Gutierrez OM, Chang Y, Shah A, Tamez H, Smith K, Thadhani R, Wolf M : Phosphorus Binders and Survival on Hemodialysis. *J. Am. Soc. Nephrol.*, 2009;20:388-396.

[37] Slatopolsky E: The intact nephron hypothesis: the concept and its implications for phosphate management in CKD-related mineral and bone disorder. *Kidney Int.,* 2011;79 (S121):3-8.

[38] O'Neill WC, Lomashvili KA: Recent progress in the treatment of vascular calcification. *Kidney Int.,* 2010;78:1232-1239.

[39] Campean V, Neureiter D, Nonnast-Daniel B et al. CD40-CD154 expression in calcified and non-calcified coronary lesions of patients with chronic renal failure. *Atherosclerosis*, 2007; 190:156–166.

[40] Blacher J, Guerin AP, Pannier B, Marchais SJ, Safar ME, London GM: Impact of aortic stiffness on survival in end-stage renal disease. *Circulation*, 1999; 99: 2434–2439.

[41] Suki W, Zabaneh R, Cangiano JL et al. Effects of sevelamer and calcium based phosphate binders on mortality in hemodialysis patients. *Kidney Int.*, 2007; 72: 1130–1137.

[42] Di Iorio B, Bellasi A, Russo D. Mortality in Kidney Disease patients Treated with Phosphate Binders: A Randomized Study. *Clin. J. Am. Soc. Nephrol.*, 2012 in press.

Index

B

D

E

F

G

H

I

J

K

L

M

N

O

P

Q

R

S

T

U

V

W

Y

Z